ACMPE Board Certification Exam Workbook

4th Edition

Published by: Medical Group Management Association (MGMA)

Library of Congress Control Number: 2020919148

Item: 1043
ISBN: 978-1-56829-060-7

Printed in the United States of America

10 9 8 7 6 5 4 3 2 1

MGMA Resources

Please note that this exam workbook provides an overview of the tasks involved in the day-to-day operations of a medical practice as detailed in the Body of Knowledge (BOK) Framework. Depending on your strengths and weaknesses, it may be advisable to explore some of these topics more thoroughly.

To that end, MGMA is constantly creating and curating resources for medical practice professionals in order to have the most up-to-date BOK in the industry. From podcasts and analysis from the nation's leading experts to tools and interactive webinars, MGMA has the knowledge you need.

Below is a partial list of the resources available at mgma.com and mgma.com/store to help direct your studies.

- **Online Education**
  - MGMA Ed
  - Webinars/Seminars
- **MGMA Data**
  - MGMA DataDive
  - Research & Analysis
  - MGMA *Stat*
- **Website Resources & Tools**
  - Certification and Fellowship
  - MGMA Career Center
  - MGMA Member Community
- **MGMA Government Affairs**
  - *Washington Connection*
- ***MGMA Connection*** **Magazine**
- **MGMA Podcasts**
  - Insights
  - Executive Session
- **MGMA Consulting**
- **Continuing Education**
- **Books**
- **Insight Articles, Member Tools, Case Studies, and More!**

Contents

Acknowledgments ... *vii*

ACMPE Continuing Education Hours ... *ix*

INTRODUCTION The Multiple-Choice and Scenario-Based Exams: Inside and Out ... 1

Test-Taking Tips ... 1

Frequently Asked Examination Questions and Tips ... 5

What is the Scenario-Based Exam Like? ... 9

Exam Preparation and Resources ... 11

CHAPTER 1 Operations Management ... 13

Task 1: General Practice Operations ... 13

Task 2: Strategic Planning ... 20

Task 3: Project Management ... 26

Task 4: Supply Chain Management and Asset Management ... 32

Task 5: Facility Management ... 38

Task 6: Business Ventures ... 47

Task 7: Information Technology ... 57

Task 8: Communications, Marketing, and Community Relations Plans ... 69

Task 9: Productivity, Compensation, and Monitoring of Benchmarks for Providers ... 81

Task 10: Quality Initiatives ... 88

Operations Management Quiz ... 94

CHAPTER 2 Financial Management ... 97

Task 1: Revenue Cycle ... 97

Task 2: Cash Flow Management ... 118

Task 3: Accounts Payable Management ... 124

Task 4: Payroll Management ... 132

Task 5: Budget Creation and Management ... 140

Task 6: Financial Reporting ... 146

Task 7: Audit Management ... 160

Task 8: Corporate Tax Reporting 165

Financial Management Quiz 177

CHAPTER 3 Human Resource Management 181

Task 1: Clinical and Nonclinical Staffing Plans 181

Task 2: Clinical and Nonclinical Staff Recruitment 185

Task 3: Labor Relations and Employment Law (Federal and State) 189

Task 4: Staff Compensation and Benefit Plans 193

Task 5: Talent Management 196

Task 6: Employee Engagement 201

Human Resource Management Quiz 204

CHAPTER 4 Transformative Healthcare Delivery 207

Task 1: Care Models 207

Task 2: Payment Models 222

Task 3: Organizational Models 228

Task 4: Innovation and Emerging Technologies 236

Transformative Healthcare Delivery Quiz 242

CHAPTER 5 Risk and Compliance Management 245

Task 1: Facilitate the Corporate Legal Structure and the Governance for the Organization 246

Task 2: Compliance with Applicable Laws and Regulations 259

Task 3: Accreditation, Credentialing, and Licensing (Individuals and Organizations) 274

Task 4: Emergency Preparedness 278

Task 5: Cybersecurity 286

Risk and Compliance Management Quiz 294

CHAPTER 6 Organizational Governance 297

Task 1: Corporate Mission, Vision, and Values 297

Task 2: Organization's Legal Structure and Governance 306

Task 3: Organizational Policy and Procedures 319

Organizational Governance Quiz 324

Acknowledgments

Thank you to the members of the ACMPE Certification Commission who guided the 2019-20 update to the Body of Knowledge for Medical Practice Management:

Tracy Bird, FACMPE, CPC, CPMA, CEMC, CPC-I
David Taylor, FACMPE, FACHE
Deborah Hudson, FACMPE
Mona Millner, MHA, NHA, FACHE, FACMPE, FHFMA, FACHCA
Andrew Smith, MHA, FACMPE
Kristina Owens, MSBA, FACMPE

Further thanks to the following MGMA members who lent their expertise as subject matter experts to update the Body of Knowledge framework and content development as memebrs of the ACMPE Body of Knowledge Oversight Committee:

Bonnie Bina, MS, MA, FACMPE
Lee Ann Webster, MA, CPA, FACMPE
Sandra Deleon, FACHE, CMPE, MSHA, MSW
Dennis Walker, CMPE, FACHE
Douglas Blackard, MHA, MS, CMPE
Eric Weaver, FACMPE, FHIMSS, FACHE
Sean Marshall, MSC, CMPE
Leland Tong, CMPE
Linda Clark, FACMPE
Amber McKinney, FACMPE
Frank Ford, MBA, MHS, FACMPE
Jeffrey Rydburg, CMPE
Cinderella Tollefsen, MBA, FACMPE
Miku Sodhi, MBBS, MD, MHA, PCMH-CCE, FACMPE
Rosalba Lozano, MBA, LSSGB, FACMPE
Andrew Smith, MHA, FACMPE
Robert Karam, BS, BSN, MA
Barbara Daniels, FACMPE
Dickson Capps, FACMPE, FACHE, FASHE, LMASCE
Dan Cole, CMPE

A special thank you is also extended to the Body of Knowledge Resource Subcomittee:

Barbara Tauscher, MHA, FACMPE
Cynthia DeCoursin, MHSA, FACMPE
Debra Ledbetter, RN, FACMPE
Judith Lento, BSH, FACMPE
Michelle Dujardin, JD, FACMPE
Frank Combs, MBA, FACMPE
Lisa Drake, RN, MBA, CMPE
Greg Davidson, MBA, FACMPE
Mary Parker, MBA, CMPE, PCMH-CCE
Susan Van der Sommen, MHA, FACHE, FACMPE
Lori Porten, CMPE
Otis C. Fagan, FACMPE
Miku Sodhi, MBBS, MD, MHA, PCMH-CCE, FACMPE
Patty Kerrins, FACMPE
Lainie Roldan, MBA, CHFP, FACMPE

A final thank you is extended to the MGMA staff and the following writers and editors for their contributions:

Penny M. Crow, MS, SHRM-SCP, RHIA *(Writer)*
Sharon Z. Ginchansky, MAOM *(Writer)*
Jim Goldmann, MHA *(Writer)*
M. Christine Kalish, MBA, CMPE *(Writer)*
Kelly Kagamas Tomkies *(Writer)*
Melissa L. Weber, MA *(Editor)*

ACMPE Continuing Education Hours

American College of Medical Practice Executives (ACMPE) participants who complete the *ACMPE Board Certification Exam Workbook* will receive four (4) hours of continuing education credit. Follow these directions to enter your credits online at www.mgma.com:

- Log in with your email address and password.
- Click on My Dashboard in the upper right-hand corner.
- Select "Manage My Account."
- Select "ACMPE Tracking" from the left navigation menu.
- Follow the instructions for "To Add Other ACMPE Continuing Education Credits ..." and select Distance Learning: Assessments for the credits type. Enter the title, the date you completed the assessment, and the four hours.

Introduction

The Multiple-Choice and Scenario-Based Exams: Inside and Out

In partial fulfillment of certification in the American College of Medical Practice Executives (ACMPE), healthcare executives seeking certification must pass both a multiple-choice examination and a scenario-based examination. These exams are developed by certified medical practice executives (CMPEs) and Fellows in the American College of Medical Practice Executives (FACMPEs) to provide a comprehensive assessment of factual information, problem-solving skills, written communication, and general management knowledge.

In this workbook introduction, each section of the exam is reviewed in detail. Test-taking tips and preparation strategies are identified, and frequently asked questions are answered. In addition, examples provide the test-taker with an accurate idea of what the questions may look like.

TEST-TAKING TIPS

Let's go over basic test-taking skills. If you've ever thought, "I'm a terrible test-taker," then these skills will be especially helpful to you. Some people might be considered naturally good at taking tests, but there's nothing stopping you from learning these skills so you can do well on tests, too.

Assess and Proceed

Board Certification through ACMPE is based on standards related to the experience of its members. The Body of Knowledge for Medical Practice Management, which provides the organizational basis for the examinations, is a living, breathing network of knowledge and skills, developed over time by professional medical practice executives. In practical terms, this means that there is no single source to refer to when preparing for the exam. As your profession develops over time, so does the Body of Knowledge and the exam.

The first step when preparing for the exam should be to assess your current level of knowledge and skills within each of the six domains in the Body of Knowledge. Most individuals will never be equally comfortable in all domains. Don't expect to know everything. Just aim for a broad understanding across all the knowledge domains and then determine a few key areas in which to focus.

This workbook provides a high-level snapshot of the knowledge and tasks contained within the Body of Knowledge as well as sample multiple-choice and essay questions and responses. The content presented here is by no means exhaustive, but once you've gone through the workbook, you should have a pretty good idea about what the exams will cover.

After assessing your current knowledge, you may decide that you are ready to take the exams. There is no substitute for just doing it. There is no penalty if you do not pass the exam. Consider taking the exam even if you don't feel 100% prepared. If you've been a practicing professional for a few years, chances are you will be familiar with most of the material and you may surprise yourself by passing without any more preparation.

Confidence

The board certification exams are experience based. This means that studying books and materials prepared by so-called experts is not the only way to prepare for the exams. It also means that by simply doing your job every day, you are developing the knowledge and skills necessary to pass the examinations.

Many of the questions are based on real-life problems and uncertainties that you confront each day. You know better than anyone that one of the best ways to learn to be a good healthcare executive is by hands-on experience. If you meet the exam prerequisite of having at least two years of experience in healthcare, chances are you have a sound knowledge base to use when taking the exam.

Think of the self-fulfilling prophecy: If you believe you will succeed, you will take actions that make success more likely. But if you tell yourself you can't achieve something, you may not have the will to prepare properly, hurting your chances of reaching your goal. If you believe you will do well on the exam, it can only help your performance.

Stress and Anxiety Management

It's important to remember that many examinees suffer from test anxiety. It's also important to know that if you surveyed CMPEs and FACMPEs, many of them would tell you that they had test anxiety. Some of them even had to take the exams more than once. But they all persisted and passed.

In the days and weeks before the test, focus on positive thoughts about the test and banish those self-doubts. It may also help to locate the testing center a few days ahead of time. This will be one less thing to worry about on the day of the test. Prepare for test day by choosing your clothing the night before and laying out other items you want to take with you. Eat healthy meals and get enough rest. Many learning experts discourage cramming or last-minute studying and, instead, advocate rest and a calm routine for best test performance. Plan to reach your testing center at least 15 minutes prior to your exam time to minimize last minute travel rush and anxiety.

There are also stress management techniques you can employ during the test itself. If you feel overwhelmed, take three deep, slow breaths. Taking a moment to center yourself and relax a little can pay off in a big way. Remember that no one question is as vital as it may seem at the time. If you aren't sure of the answer, you can come back to the question later.

Overcoming Test Anxiety

Test anxiety is an uneasiness or apprehension experienced before, during, or after an examination because of concern, worry, or fear. Almost everyone experiences some anxiety.

What Can Be Done About It?

Fortunately, there is a great deal that you can do to keep the anxiety from interfering with your performance. First, it's important to know that you don't have to eliminate it entirely. It helps to be up for exams. You just want to reduce the anxiety to a manageable level.

Getting prepared for the exam is more than half the battle. Reading this workbook is a great step to ensure you know what is expected of you. Take the practice tests and use the available support materials. The results will help guide you to where you should concentrate any study efforts. Use a method such as survey, question, read, recite, review for reading your related materials. Make flashcards and review them often. If necessary, make outlines and summary sheets. Ask yourself, "What is the important information?"

How Do You Become Self-Confident?

Use positive self-talk. Research shows that the self-talk of test-anxious people almost always tends to be negative and self-defeating: "Everyone is smarter and faster than I am." "I always mess up on tests." "These are trick questions."

Become aware of what you say to yourself. Try writing your negative thoughts and then disputing each one with a positive statement. Start to encourage yourself as you would a friend. Repeating positive statements to yourself will help reprogram your mind for success instead of failure.

Before the exams:

- Visualize yourself doing well and reaching your goal of certification.
- Try not to compare yourself with others.
- Become an expert in learning what is going well and what you can do to improve. Collect data by keeping a journal.
- Reward yourself after studying instead of getting involved in avoidance behaviors.
- Practice relaxing (progressive relaxation, self-hypnosis, guided imagery, etc.) so that relaxation becomes an automatic response.
- Aim for a state of relaxed concentration. When you concentrate, you have all of your energy focused on your work and none wasted on worry.
- Take care of yourself by eating well and getting enough sleep.
- Plan time to exercise regularly — and do it.

During the exams:

- Read the directions, plan your approach, and schedule your time.
- Carefully read each question, flagging those that you would like to return to later.
- Focus your attention on the test. Don't waste time and energy worrying, thinking about the consequences of not doing well, or wondering what others are doing.
- Suggest to yourself that you probably know the correct answer and the answer will come to you when you get back to it. Note that you are not penalized for incorrect answers.
- If you start to feel anxious, practice your relaxation techniques. Use anxiety as a cue to relax. Close your eyes, take three deep breaths, and then move back to the task.

For both exams, study practical situations a healthcare executive faces every day. *MGMA Connection* articles, member-benefit webinars, and conversations on the MGMA Community pages are a great place to start. The questions are designed to focus on critical skills/knowledge that a candidate would be expected to show in real-life situations. You are encouraged to solicit input from CMPEs and FACMPEs.

For the scenario-based exam, read each paragraph carefully to make sure you understand what the scenario is presenting and process all important information. Do not try to answer the questions prior to reading and understanding the scenario.

For the multiple-choice exam, think of your own answer before looking at the choices provided. Eliminate clearly wrong answers. After you have answered those you know, return to those you checked. Think about only one question at a time.

If your time is running out, concentrate on those questions you know well. Use all the time allowed for reviewing your answers and completing ideas. Only change answers if you are sure of yourself.[1]

Pace Yourself

Question design is not a mystery or a grand attempt to stump you; we want you to pass this exam. Questions and answers are researched individually and reviewed by a subject matter expert. In the next two sections, we discuss a few more scenario-based and multiple-choice test-taking skills. By learning and practicing these skills, you will increase your chance for success. You can adopt a new attitude of "I'm a great test-taker."

For the multiple-choice exam, you will have 195 minutes to answer 175 questions. You have more than a minute per question; this may not sound like much, but most examinees have more than enough time not only to answer each question, but also to check their answers before completing the test.

The scenario-based exam begins with a paragraph describing a typical situation in a healthcare executive's daily life. Each scenario will require you to define the appropriate steps that should be followed to resolve the issues. The test will include 18 to 25 scenarios and require you to make choices from three to five items in each set, equaling approximately 90 total items. You will have 120 minutes to complete this section.

FREQUENTLY ASKED EXAMINATION QUESTIONS AND TIPS

Who writes the exam questions?

Exam questions are created by the ACMPE Examinations Committee, Exam Development Committee, and Exam Development Committee writers. These volunteers are experienced healthcare executives from varied professional backgrounds who are committed to advancing the professional growth of their peers. These members represent medical practices of different sizes, specialties, and governance structures from throughout the United States. The writers are selected in this way to fairly represent the broad spectrum of professional settings in which healthcare executives work. Exam questions are developed to represent this broad national standard.

How are the exam questions written?

Questions for both exams are drafted by individual committee members, then reviewed by at least one other subject matter expert and one item development expert. Then, these questions are reviewed by the full Examination Committee, which discusses the best wording before proofreading and final approval from the psychometrician's development team. Questions are evaluated to ensure that they are understandable, written to comply with best practice in item-writing, and focused on current practices within the profession.

How does MGMA ensure that exam questions are fair and valid?

After the Examinations Committee approves a question, it is added to a bank of questions organized by the categories within the Body of Knowledge for Medical Practice Management. The question bank provides a pool of possible exam questions.

The performance of the exam questions is evaluated by psychometric consultants. Statistical results from each question on this exam are evaluated to determine whether they meet certification standards for validity and fairness. In addition, the statistical performance of the exam as a whole is evaluated to determine whether it meets predetermined standards for validity. Questions that display questionable statistical properties are reviewed by the Examinations Committee, which determines whether to score them and include them in future exams or not to include them in examinee scores and to revise the item for future evaluation.

In addition to the psychometric review process, the entire exam item bank is periodically reviewed by the Examinations Committee to ensure that questions remain up to date. If a question is determined to be statistically invalid or out of date, it is retired. Actual exam questions will never appear in practice exams or sample questions.

How are questions within the multiple-choice exam organized?

Every question in the exam item bank is identified by its place within the Body of Knowledge for Medical Practice Management. The questions on the multiple-choice exam for each knowledge domain from the Body of Knowledge are weighted according to their importance and frequency, as determined during the job task analysis conducted.

The percentage of questions for each knowledge domain is organized as shown in Exhibit 0.1.

How are the exams scored?

MGMA uses a professional testing partner to score the multiple-choice and scenario-based exams. One point is granted for each correct answer of a multiple-choice item (choose 1), and partial credit is given for each multi-select item (choose 2 or 3). There is no penalty assessed for an incorrect answer; points are scored only for correct answers. The number of questions answered correctly (or total points) is a candidate's raw score.

A candidate's raw score is converted to a scaled score, which is similar to scores provided for college entrance exams. The total scaled score will determine whether a candidate has passed the exam. This scaled score is statistically derived from the candidate's raw score and can range from 200 to 800. The passing scaled score for the exam is 500. The passing score reflects the minimum amount of knowledge a committee of experts has determined to be appropriate for certification, according to established standard-setting practices.

EXHIBIT 0.1
Questions per Knowledge Domain

Knowledge Domain	Percent of Exam	Number of Multiple-Choice Questions	Number of Scenario-Based Questions
Operations Management	25	43	22
Financial Management	25	44	23
Human Resource Management	15	26	14
Transformative Healthcare Delivery	13	23	12
Risk and Compliance Management	12	21	11
Organizational Governance	10	18	8

MGMA, like many testing programs, uses multiple test forms to limit exposure of test questions. As new forms of the exams are introduced, a certain number of questions in each content area are replaced by new questions. While the new questions measure the same content as the questions they replace, it is very rare that they are of the same level of difficulty. These changes may cause one form of the exam to be slightly more or less difficult than another form.

To adjust for these differences in difficulty, a statistical procedure called *equating* is used. The goal of equating is to ensure fairness to all candidates. In the equating process, the minimum raw score (number of correctly answered questions) required to equal the passing raw score on the base form is statistically determined. For example, if the exam is determined to be more difficult than the base form of the exam, then the minimum raw score required to pass will be slightly lower than the passing scaled score. If the exam is a bit easier, then the passing raw score will be slightly higher than the passing raw score on the base form. Equating helps ensure that the passing scaled score represents the same level of knowledge, regardless of which form of the exam a candidate takes. Finally, these raw scores are translated into the common scale so that the same scale score represents the passing standard on both forms.

As the test is a criterion-referenced test, or one that compares performance against an established criterion as described earlier, your passing status is not determined by the performance of other candidates.

Note: The passing point set for the exam cannot be appealed. To score one point below the passing point is to be unsuccessful on the exam; to score at the passing point or higher is to pass the exam. A score higher than the passing point is not an indication of a higher proficiency in the subject matter. Because of exam confidentiality, it is MGMA's policy to disclose neither the values of the score bandwidths nor which questions were answered incorrectly.

Will I be penalized for wrong answers?

You will not be penalized for wrong answers. The exam score is calculated using only the number of questions you answered correctly out of the total scorable questions. This means that unanswered or wrong answers do not count against you. For this reason, it is best to guess on a question you are unsure of because unanswered questions will never gain you a point, but a guess might be correct. The process of elimination will aid in this method and is discussed later.

When will I find out if I passed the exams?

Exam results are immediate and can be shown after exam completion, or in the score portal after completion.

What happens if I do not pass the exams?

If you do not pass the multiple-choice or scenario-based exam, the score portal will provide your overall score and feedback by knowledge domain. This study aid can help you to focus on those areas where you may need additional knowledge to pass the exam.

Exam results are independent of each other. If you pass the scenario-based exam but do not pass the multiple-choice portion, you will only need to retake the multiple-choice exam.

What are the multiple-choice questions like?

The multiple-choice questions have four answer options and one correct answer. Some test items are explanation or definition questions; others require application of the topic in question. Here are two sample questions to review.

1. **Which step of Six Sigma involves gathering data about each step of the process being improved?**

   A. Define

   B. Measure

   C. Analyze

   D. Control

2. **How should all projects that use project management be closed?**

   A. By having a final project meeting

   B. By conducting surveys

   C. By completing a written report

   D. By identifying total project costs

The first question asks you to define a business concept. The second question asks you how everyday business concepts are handled in the workplace. While there are some definition or explanation questions on the objective exam, most questions will ask you to apply your knowledge to a practice setting.

WHAT IS THE SCENARIO-BASED EXAM LIKE?

The scenario-based exam consists of 18 to 25 sets, each presenting a scenario followed by three to four questions that focus on critical skills/knowledge that a candidate would be expected to show in the described situation and are drawn from the six domains. Each scenario set starts with a set header of an incident that may occur in a practice, or a summary of problems presented to a healthcare executive to handle. Following each set are 3 to 5 items pertaining to the scenario prompt in either multiple-choice, multi-select, or drag-and-drop item types. The answers either help in the action plan, give greater detail on what the problem is proposing, or identify what needs to be evaluated to assess the situation.

USE THE FOLLOWING SCENARIO TO ANSWER PRACTICE QUESTIONS 1-4

You are the executive of an established physician practice of 10 physicians. In their meetings, the group has discussed a desire to expand in and add a location in a new adjoining market. Through market connections, you have found an existing external group of three (3) physicians who would like to join your group. However, your physician leader just recently shared that he is now hearing that not all physicians are excited about growth.

1. What action step should you perform first?

A. Meet with each physician individually to discuss their perspective

B. Call an emergency meeting of the group to discuss

C. Complete a financial analysis for adding a location

D. Review social and economic demographics of the new adjoining market

Answer: B

2. What are ways to strengthen the group's decision-making, resulting in increased unity on the growth decisions? – CHOOSE TWO

A. Create forum for open dialogue and sharing of perspectives in group meetings

B. Only discuss topic if at least six of the 10 physicians are present in group meetings

C. Hold a planning retreat once a year to discuss growth

D. Review a business plan for the new growth in a group meeting

E. Hold the group meeting at 6 p.m.

Answer: A, D

3. **If the group decides to move forward, what actions should be completed as part of credentialing?**
– CHOOSE THREE

A. Ensure the group and new physicians are a good cultural fit

B. Query the National Practitioner Data Bank

C. Complete Primary Source Verification

D. Check OIG sanctions exclusion database

E. Ensure current professional liability insurance is occurrence-based

Answer: B, C, D

Tips for the Exams

Read the Questions Carefully

It is easy to feel rushed on any exam. If you begin to hurry through the questions, remind yourself that only giving the questions a cursory glance is not much better than not finishing the exam. Chances are, you will be able to finish the exam with time to spare, so be sure to read the questions carefully. When in a hurry, it can be easy to read a question the wrong way. Be sure you fully understand what the question is asking before moving on to your answer choices.

Give All the Responses a Chance

It is best to read over all of the answer choices before choosing your answer. The test instructions tell you to choose the best answer. This means that there could be one partially right answer and another answer that more fully or better fits the question asked. Even if the first answer option looks good, read all the way through the other options before making your choice.

Use the Process of Elimination

As discussed in the last section, you are not penalized for wrong answers. But you are rewarded for correct answers, so the more of those you get, the better. If you must make a blind guess, either because you are running out of time or because you do not know the answer, you have a 25% chance of choosing the correct answer. However, if you can read through the four choices and see one that absolutely cannot be correct, eliminate it. You now have a 33% chance of guessing the right answer. Sometimes you can even eliminate two options and increase your chances of guessing correctly up to 50%.

EXAM PREPARATION AND RESOURCES

The most effective way to prepare for the exams is to do your job every day. If you are working within a large system where specific departments handle individual functions such as human resources, make it a point to ask questions and get to know the experts in your own organization. If you work in a small organization, quiz your accountant or attorney about why they are making the recommendations they provide to you and what resources they would suggest to increase your understanding of the particular issues that you are working on at the time.

Get to know other members in the certification program through local or state MGMA chapters by attending MGMA conferences in person or virtually, or by joining online member communities. Other members can become your best resource to answer specific questions and link you to sources of information to aid in your test preparation. Some areas have local face-to-face study groups that meet to support each other through the certification process. In addition, there are online study groups available through the MGMA member community.

Once you've identified the areas where you want to focus your study, there are many resources to aid in your preparation. Hundreds of articles on practice-related topics from MGMA publications are available as a benefit to members on mgma.com. Members can easily search the website for any article that has appeared in our publications, ACMPE Fellowship papers, and other resources.

Finally, there are a number of seminars, books, surveys, tools, and online courses available through MGMA, as well as other organizations, which may aid in your study of particular topics.

We wish you the best of luck and hope you'll stay in touch!

Note

1. B. Probert, *Test Anxiety* (Gainesville, FL: University of Florida Counseling Center, 2003), www.counseling.ufl.edu/cwc/uploads/docs/Academic%20Concerns/Test%20Anxiety.pdf.

Chapter 1

Operations Management

Operations management in a medical practice includes planning, purchasing materials and equipment, managing and maintaining facilities, forging business partnerships, and creating marketing and communication plans.

How do you develop and implement an effective business plan? How do you ensure the effective management of day-to-day operations? The key knowledge and tasks necessary to effectively manage business operations are:

1. General Practice Operations
2. Strategic Planning
3. Project Management
4. Supply Chain Management and Asset Management
5. Facility Management
6. Business Ventures
7. Information Technology
8. Communications, Marketing, and Community Relations Plans
9. Productivity, Compensation, and Monitoring of Benchmarks for Providers
10. Quality Initiatives

TASK 1: GENERAL PRACTICE OPERATIONS

General practice operations are defined and guided by policies and procedures that ensure patients are scheduled accurately and quickly, patient wait times and visits are efficient and effective, and patients receive quality healthcare and accurate communications. In order to accomplish these goals, it is necessary to know what the industry benchmarks are in each of these areas, apply total quality management techniques to initiate needed improvements, and then create or revise policies and procedures that communicate these improvements to all staff.

1.1 Industry Benchmarks

One of the most important tasks a medical practice can complete is gathering appropriate industry benchmarks and measuring the same items at their practice. Benchmarks allow the healthcare executive to understand industry trends in important areas to see where the practice could improve. Practices should be using both internal and external benchmarks. In other words, the healthcare executive should be comparing how the practice is doing from one month to the next, and from one year to the next, to recognize any trends that may be of concern.

There are a few reliable sources of benchmarking data available for practices today. They include:

- Medical Group Management Association (MGMA)
- American Medical Association, Division of Economic and Health Policy Research
- American Health Information Management Association
- Healthcare Billing and Management Association
- Your practice's billing service

Medical practices can use this data to determine if their performance in many areas of operations is in line with the performance of other practices. For example, if the practice's wait time is much longer than other, similar practices' wait time, the practice should look at ways to improve that process.

The most commonly used benchmarks are:

- **Provider productivity:** There are many factors that contribute to provider productivity. They include the number of physicians, the number of nurse practitioners, the percentage of time they spend in patient care, provider support (i.e., do providers have the space, equipment, etc., they need?), number of scheduled patients, number of work hours per provider, etc. Another measure of productivity was first introduced by the Centers for Medicare and Medicaid Services (CMS): relative value unit, or RVU.
- **Provider compensation:** Provider compensation benchmarks include total salary with bonuses and incentives, retirement dollars, and any other compensation received.
- **Non-provider compensation:** Non-provider compensation includes total salary, any bonuses or incentives, and any money going into retirement savings accounts. This dollar amount can be used to compare to other practices' non-provider compensation, and in determining other benchmarks.

- **Non-provider staffing:** This benchmark looks at the number of staff members working at the practice who are not providing patient care.
- **Patient experience:** Practices can collect benchmarking data on patient experience by inviting patients to complete surveys after their encounters with providers.
- **Reputation management:** Reputation management refers to the attitudes about the practice in the media, and especially reviews the practice receives online through social media sites. Both positive and negative reviews should be tracked, data collected on the ratio of positive to negative reviews, and the reviews analyzed for patterns or trends.
- **No-shows:** No-shows are patients who do not keep scheduled appointments.
- **Patient access:** Patient access refers to whether the practice's patients or potential patients can schedule appointments at their convenience, if the type of care they require is available, and if healthcare is affordable.
- **Turnover:** Turnover in medical practices refers to how long providers and non-providers stay and work at medical practices.
- **Quality:** Practices can find quality benchmarks through the Healthcare Effectiveness Data and Information Set (HEDIS), Merit-based Incentive Payment System (MIPS), and the Medicare Access and CHIP Reauthorization Act (MACRA) system.
- **Rate of Readmission:** This rate is determined by tracking the number of patients who are released by the hospital and then readmitted for treatment for the same or a related health concern within 30 days.

1.2 Total Quality Management Techniques

KEY TERMS

Lean: Lean is a fundamental change in how people within an organization think and what they value, thus transforming how they behave.

Six Sigma: Six Sigma is a continuous approach, which means the organization never stops using it to improve processes. Six Sigma is a set of tools and a methodology for process improvement, based on gathering data and statistics.

Total quality management (TQM): TQM seeks to integrate an organization's functions with respect to meeting customer needs and organizational objectives. TQM subscribes to the principles of doing the right thing the first time and every time and looking at quality as a constantly moving target.

Both Six Sigma and Lean are techniques for improving the effectiveness, efficiency, and quality of business processes. These techniques were first used to improve efficiencies in manufacturing processes, but they were broadened to include any business process in any type of industry. In the healthcare setting, both approaches can be integrated and used to improve the efficiency, effectiveness, and quality of patient care.

Six Sigma uses a five-step approach:

1. **Define**: Define the problem or process you want to improve and set measurable goals for improvement
2. **Measure**: Measure how the process is currently performing and gather data at each step in the process
3. **Analyze**: Analyze the data you gathered and use it to identify ways to improve, such as eliminating bottlenecks
4. **Improve**: Develop and test solutions or improvements
5. **Control**: After solutions or improvements have been implemented, continue to monitor or measure the process to ensure it has been improved and continues to work better

The basic principles of Lean are to:

- **Specify value**: Your practice must determine which activities or services offered and provided every day are of value to your patients, that is, value-added activities and services that are necessary to patients and for which they are willing to pay
- **Engage the staff**: This is best accomplished through training
- **Eliminate waste**: The process of eliminating problems, such as overproduction, long patient wait times, extra work for staff that serves no purpose, and motion waste
- **Create patient access**: Refers to the ability to respond to customer demand

There are many tools that your practice can use as it completes the Lean Six Sigma process. Here are a few you may want to consider using, depending on your practice's goals and the processes being improved:

- Value stream mapping is a lean tool that uses a flowchart to map each step of a process.
- A fishbone diagram is used to uncover the cause and effect of a specific problem.
- A Kanban System allows practices to visualize the flow of work and processes. It includes all aspects of a particular process including the supply chain of materials.
- A Pareto chart shows trends in a process or type of work over time.
- A swimlane chart is used to map the flow of work to the people responsible for doing it.

- A RACI chart is used to ensure that each step of the implementation occurs when it needs to. Each step of the implementation process should be assigned to a specific person.

Once the practice has determined solutions to the problems or identified new procedures that need to be implemented to improve a process or workflow, the work does not end there. Monitoring and measuring the new process to ensure it is working as planned is important. Measurement and review will demonstrate that the change has improved the flow or solved the problem. Monitoring the new process regularly also ensures that the gains the practice receives from the changes are maintained.

Staff members who lead or regularly take part in the practice's process improvement efforts should receive training in the Lean Six Sigma techniques. Training can take place through ASQ or several other organizations.

1.3 Policies and Procedures

Healthcare executives are responsible for creating and maintaining policies and procedures that keep practice operations moving efficiently. If there are no policies and procedures in place for all providers and staff members to follow, employees are unclear about their place in the organization and how their job should be performed.

Health information management (HIM) policies have become increasingly important. HIPAA standards and other government guidelines have led the industry to use electronic health records, or EHRs. Electronic health records are more accessible to providers, patients' insurance companies and patients themselves.

The American Health Information Management Association (AHIMA) recommends these best practices when it comes to HIM policies:

- Review existing policies and procedures, including workflows and internal actions.
- Establish a HIPAA structure for provider relations. This means if your practice works with other healthcare providers, you should create a written and signed agreement that outlines how, when, and why health information will be shared.
- Review HIM compliance practices on a regular basis.
- Manage patient consent policies and practices to ensure compliance with regulations.
- Manage access to protected health information (PHI) to ensure your practice's policies and procedures comply with government privacy rules.
- Create and provide a standardized consent form to share PHI and EHR.[1]

Patient scheduling is a complex topic with many areas of concern. Practices should consider their patients when determining how to schedule visits and procedures. Patient cycle time is also a concern. This is the time it takes from patient check-in until the patient checks out. Patient cycle time is usually 1.5 times the amount of time the patient spends with the provider. Cycle time is a factor for measuring patient satisfaction, included with the overall time spent in patient care at a medical practice

The next most important factor to consider is the medical practice's throughput. This means, from the time the patient enters the office until the time they leave, how smoothly and efficiently does the visit flow? Practices should consider the following when examining their throughput. These are processes that should be benchmarked and measured to look for opportunities for improvement:

- Length of time between appointment time and roomed time
- Length of time between patient roomed to physician entry
- Length of time the physician is in the room
- Total time between the appointment time and the time the patient leaves
- Late patients — how many minutes are they late, and how do they affect the schedule?
- Appointments abandoned — how many times does this occur and why?
- Patient communication — How much communication takes place throughout the visit, and how long does each conversation take?

Gaps in care and patient compliance are related to HEDIS, or the Healthcare Effectiveness Data and Information Set produced by the National Committee for Quality Assurance (NCQA). HEDIS is used by more than 90% of U.S. health plans to measure quality of care. HEDIS uses 90 measures across five domains of care to evaluate quality of care. During this process, gaps in care are identified. When gaps in care and patient compliance are identified, it is important to communicate with staff members and create or revise existing policies or procedures to improve quality.

Reputation management also has become a critical factor of a medical practice's success. Practices must manage their online reputation in order to succeed in the market.

Referral management refers to two processes: outbound referrals, and inbound referrals. Outbound referrals are offered by providers within the practice for patients who need more specialized care, tests, or procedures not offered by the practice. Your practice should have a system in place for noting these referrals to ensure patients make the appointments with the other providers. The practice should know whether their patient choses a different provider or did not get the recommended procedure. Inbound referrals are those made by other providers recommending your practice or a specific physician at your practice. Your practice should be tracking where referrals come from, how quickly these patients make appointments once referred, the percentage of patients referred who made appointments, and why patients who were referred chose not to schedule an appointment.

It is important to review and update all of the practice's policies and procedures on a regular basis. That means assigning the most appropriate staff members to review each type of policy, and scheduling the review at the same time each year.

SAMPLE QUESTIONS

1. **Why should medical practices use benchmarks?**

   A. They allow the healthcare executive to understand industry trends in important areas to see where the practice could improve

   B. They allow the healthcare executive to recognize when staff members in the practice are not performing well

   C. They allow the healthcare executive to understand why the practice may be struggling financially

   D. They allow the healthcare executive to recognize industry trends in healthcare to see additional services the practice could add

2. **Why are total quality management techniques such as Lean and Six Sigma used in medical practices?**

   A. To engage the staff

   B. To reduce practice turnover

   C. To improve the efficiency, effectiveness, and quality of patient care

   D. To expand patient services

Answers: 1-A, 2-C

TASK 2: STRATEGIC PLANNING

Strategic planning is an ongoing process of organizational change, described as "a disciplined effort to produce fundamental decisions and actions that shape and guide what an organization is, what it does, and why it does it, with a focus on the future."[2]

Strategic planning in today's changing times has become extremely important for a practice. It focuses on longer-term goals and strategy rather than just short-term objectives. This important process will allow all stakeholders to have a clear understanding of the direction of the organization. Planning is required when the future state we desire involves a set of interdependent decisions, that is, a system of decisions.[3]

The key knowledge necessary to effectively develop and implement strategic plans includes:

- Identify organizational goals and needs
- Set goals and assign responsibility
- Align business plans with the mission and strategy of the organization
- Monitor the effectiveness of the plans

2.1 Role of Mission and Vision in the Strategic Management Process

KEY TERMS

Mission: The organization's purpose or reason for being is usually illustrated in a mission statement.

Vision: The vision statement of an organization outlines what an organization wants to be. It is future-oriented, inspirational, and ambitious; however, it is also realistic and achievable.

Core values: Core values represent the core priorities in the organization's culture, including what beliefs drive members and how they truly act in the organization.

Strategic objectives: Strategic objectives are tactical, mid- to short-term actions that are taken to accomplish a goal.

The first step in the strategic planning process is to define the medical group practice's mission. If the practice cannot clearly articulate its purpose, its values, and the direction it is headed, then the remaining steps in the planning process cannot be addressed. In other words, all planning for the organization hinges on the mission statement.

- The mission is the organization's precise statement of purpose
- It describes why the organization exists
- It helps keep management focused on preserving or strengthening the organization's unique competitive niche

- It helps transform ideas into action
- It can also prevent panic and unwise marketing or spending responses to meet an indirect threat by competitors
- Most organizations have limited resources, and a mission statement is a constant reminder of where those limited resources should be focused

Typically, a vision is "more important as a guide to implementing strategy than it is to formulating it."[4] This is because strategy development is driven by what the organization is trying to accomplish, which is the organization's purpose. A vision is more encompassing than the mission. It answers the question: What does the organization look like as it effectively carries out its mission? It is the pursuit of this image of success that really motivates people to work together.

Values represent the organization's highest priorities and deeply held driving forces. They are statements about how the organization will value customers, suppliers, and the internal community. Value statements describe actions that are the living enactment of the fundamental values held by most individuals within the organization. Values are increasingly important in strategic planning, often driving the intent and direction for the planning team.[5]

The coordination and facilitation of strategic planning in general should be designated as the responsibility of a key stakeholder, and development of the strategy should be in line with each stakeholder responsible. They should understand the strategic implications of their decisions.[6] The rationale for this is that the managers and staff members are more in touch with the activities that take place within their areas because they are firsthand responders. Who better to identify areas of change than those who have identified the need for it?

Once the facilitator has been determined, the strategic planning team should be formed. The first step in establishing the team is to identify its membership. For example, determine who will be directly involved in planning, who will provide key information to the process, who will review the plan, who will authorize the plan, and who will lead implementation of the plan. There should be at least one person appointed to the team who ultimately has authority to make strategic decisions (i.e., to select which goals will be achieved and how). The composition of the team also should ensure that as many stakeholders as possible, both internal and external, are involved in the planning process. They should be from all areas of the organization and have various backgrounds and points of views. Internal stakeholders, such as physicians and clinical and clerical staff members, should be well represented. Each will bring a different perspective to the process. External stakeholders, such as patients and contract staff members, may have valuable input at some point in the planning process, so it is a good idea to include them when appropriate. Exercise caution, because many of these external stakeholders may also share this type of relationship with the organization's competitors. Sometimes, it may be wise to communicate the confidentiality of meetings and possibly ask participants to sign nondisclosure agreements.

The next step is to determine the optimal number of meetings the committee should have and the timeline for gathering information, assessing the data, and writing the plan.

The final step in the planning-to-plan process is to provide the team with the tools and resources it needs to develop, implement, and maintain the plan. Adequate resources in the form of supplies (white board, markers, flipcharts, paper, etc.), time, money, and creative freedom need to be dedicated to this task. If this is a new undertaking within the organization, funds should be dedicated to hiring a facilitator or consultant, or sending staff to training.

A medical practice needs to evaluate exactly where it is in the market before it can determine what steps to take to achieve its goals. To do this, the strategic management team will need to undertake an analysis of the practice and its current place in the market. The team also needs to analyze the market itself, as well as identify current and future opportunities. All of this requires the practice to gather relevant, meaningful data. This step can include conducting a SWOT analysis, collecting data, identifying business drivers, and analyzing the data collected.

A strengths, weaknesses, opportunities, and threats (SWOT) analysis can help the organization assess the internal environment (strengths and weaknesses) and external environment (opportunities and threats). The SWOT process involves several steps and is often conducted in the context of a group meeting or retreat.

The two key questions a SWOT analysis addresses are:

1. What are the significant issues that the group practice faces today?
2. How should the group practice attend to these issues?

EXHIBIT 1.1

Strategic Plan SWOT Analysis

INTERNAL FACTORS	EXTERNAL FORCES
Strengths	**Opportunities**
What does your practice do well? In this cell, the internal strengths of the practice should be highlighted. Strengths can relate to the practice at large, to the environment, to perceptions, and to people. "People" elements include the skills, capabilities, and knowledge of participants.	***Where are the opportunities for your practice?*** In this cell, the external opportunities for the practice should be highlighted. Opportunities can entail socioeconomic, environmental, and demographic factors.
Weaknesses	**Threats**
What part of your practice needs improvement? In this cell, the internal weaknesses of the practice are identified. This should include an honest appraisal of how things are in the practice. It is not uncommon for "people" problems to emerge as major weaknesses (e.g., poor communication, lack of leadership, little trust, etc.).	***What is happening in your area that could threaten your practice?*** In this cell, the external threats for the practice are identified. Threats are events that may, with a change of emphasis or perception, adversely affect the practice. The same factors may emerge as both a threat and an opportunity.

Collecting objective data will streamline the decision-making ability of healthcare professionals during the strategic planning process. Setting standards for how this data should be collected is important so that decision-makers can have a picture of what is occurring across the organization. There are four steps for successful data and information gathering:

1. Begin with the end result in mind. Understand what the team and its charter aim to accomplish. Careful planning will prevent unneeded data collection. All data collected should clearly contribute to the outcome.
2. Before data collection begins, document the assumptions and methodology for collection. For example, if exam room utilization needs to be determined, you will need to answer and document the following questions:
    - Will extra time be allowed for room turnover?
    - Will lunch hours be included in the data?
    - How will seasonal variation be accounted for?
3. Communicate your goals. Key stakeholders need to understand the methodology and assumptions in data collection before they begin. Identify those stakeholders early. If key people don't buy into your methodology and assumptions, they might not trust the objective data you are working to collect. When considering stakeholders, remember frontline staff. The data collection often will involve unusual activity in the clinical area. Make sure staff members know why unfamiliar people might be in their workspaces. You might also want to leverage staff to collect certain types of data.
4. Collect the data and analyze it based on the assumptions you made at the beginning of the process.

Once the data has been collected, perform a detailed analysis of it so the team can understand the environment and determine where the practice needs to go.

A number of methods to analyze costs, benefits, and risks are associated with any decision or plan, including cost-benefit analysis and group self-assessment.

Cost-Benefit Analysis

The procedure always involves the following steps:

1. Define the plan or the decision and the process by drawing a flowchart or by listing all inputs, outputs, activities, and events, using the budget or other financial statements and information as guides
2. Calculate the cost and benefit of each service (include, if possible, direct, indirect, financial, and social costs and benefits)
3. Compare the sum of the costs with the sum of the benefits
4. Select the best choices if alternatives are being considered

Ultimately, the most significant resources of the group practice are the providers. Facilities are useless without the clinical staff to perform services. The specialty areas of training of the providers limit and define the scope of services offered to the community. The practice should acknowledge the importance of the providers by conducting a confidential internal survey.

Once the strategic plan is final and ready to be implemented, it needs to be shared with key stakeholders and staff. Communication should be ongoing as the plan is developed, with regular updates delivered to key stakeholders. Once the plan is complete, it should be shared with the wider practice members as well. An implementation plan should also be shared.

To maximize the benefits of engagement of all stakeholders, leaders in the strategic planning process need to communicate often. All employees should be aware of the practice's mission, vision, values, goals and objectives. All stakeholders should be kept informed of the planning team's status and progress. Physicians should be considered key stakeholders, and special effort should be made to ensure they are engaged with the strategic planning process. Healthcare executives need to involve physician input from the beginning. The healthcare executive needs to plan for the planning process.

In addition to being informed of the strategic plan, stakeholders should be invited to take ownership of a part of the plan's implementation. Whether it is stakeholders, other key leaders or staff members who take ownership, each part of the strategic plan should have an owner who is responsible for implementing that part. The team should continue to meet and discuss implementation efforts and any issues that may arise. Monitoring should also include:

- Ensuring activities are within the parameters of the plan
- Making sure activities are consistent with the practice's mission, vison, and goals
- Continuing to review internal and external changes, such as new legislation, which may affect the strategic plan

SAMPLE QUESTIONS

1. **What is the first step in the strategic planning process?**

   A. Select a facilitator

   B. Define the practice's mission

   C. Collect data

   D. Perform analysis

2. **How does a medical practice evaluate where it is in the market?**

   A. Define the practice's mission

   B. Communicate the strategic plan

   C. Survey the community

   D. Undertake an analysis of the practice and its current place in the market

Answers: 1-B, 2-D

TASK 3: PROJECT MANAGEMENT

Managing a medical practice is a complex task. Constantly changing regulations, electronic medical health records, technologies, insurance models, and many other changes make managing the practice a challenging undertaking. Using project management techniques allows the healthcare executive to implement needed updates and changes in an organized, methodical way that gives these changes a better chance for success.

KEY TERM

SMART goals: Goals that are specific, measurable, achievable, realistic, and timely, or tangible.

3.1 Tactics

The first decision you will need to make is whether a project requires the use of formal project management processes or not. Especially when you are pressed for time, you may be tempted to abandon a more organized approach to projects, but this may be the best time to engage project management methods. Small, short-term projects may not require full implementation, but will benefit from some methods. Once you have decided the level of project management methods that will be engaged, it is time to initiate the project and establish its goals.

Initiating the project involves the following steps:[7]

- Define the scope of the project
- Develop specific goals
- Define key project milestones
- Define deliverables
- Outline tasks (and determine responsible person for each task)
- Determine costs
- Establish deadlines

Project initiation will involve doing some research in order to complete all of the above tasks. Research could include finding background information and completing market research. Extensive research needs could be included as one of the project goals.

Team members should include:

- Project manager
- Project sponsor
- Subject matter experts
- Managers in charge of resources
- Staff members involved in the process or product

Use SMART goals. By using SMART goals, you avoid the mistakes of making goals too broad, vague, or undefined. Each proposed project goal should meet these criteria before it becomes part of the project.

During the planning phase, you create a step-by-step plan for executing the project. Planning should be transparent, which means all team members, stakeholders, and the project sponsor should clearly see that the plan is designed to meet the goals and there are no hidden objectives.

A critical part of the project plan is the project schedule, which should be reasonable and allow the team to see the flow of work, progress and deadlines. The team should also develop and adhere to a communication plan that will ensure the team communicates with the appropriate people on a regular basis. To do this, the project management team needs to identify the audiences that need to be informed of the progress of the project.

The project plan should contain a comprehensive list of all the resources that are needed to complete the project, including any staff members who need to participate.

Tracking the progress of the project is an important part of its execution. Tracking allows the team to see progress and make changes if things begin to go askew. Changes can be made before too much time is lost. Tracking also gives the team the ability to ensure that regulations are being followed.

There are a number of project management tools your practice can use to implement its project plans. The most commonly used include Gantt charts, shared file sites, and flowcharts and diagrams. A Gantt chart is a specific type of spreadsheet that is designed to help project managers stay on top of data, assignments, and the overall flow of projects (see example in Figure 1.1).

Figure 1.1[8]

[Project Name] [Company Name] [Project Manager]						**Week 1**							**Week 2**							**Week 3**						
Task Name	**Task Owner**	**Start Date**	**End Date**	**Duration**	**Progress**	M	T	W	T	F	S	S	M	T	W	T	F	S	S	M	T	W	T	F	S	S
[Task]	[Name]	[Date]	[Date]	[# of Days]	[%]																					

Throughout the course of a project, team members will need to share files and project information. Some documents are living documents, meaning they are open to comments and changes from team members, or they will need to be updated frequently. Using shared file sites such as SharePoint, Microsoft Teams, and Google Drive gives team members the ability to share files and information instantly among all team members.

Flowcharts and diagrams are other common project management tools. In general, a process flowchart can be used for large, complex processes so team members can visualize how the project will flow. A flowchart can be helpful when different staff members or departments are involved at different stages of the project.

Part of the project management process is establishing risks and boundaries. This should occur in the planning phase and be reassessed as needed as things change throughout the project. Risks means threats that could affect the success of the project, as well as the risks that are naturally associated with the successful completion of the project. For example, the practice may launch a project to purchase, install, and train employees on new diagnostic equipment.

Project boundaries can be defined as the predetermined limitations of the project, such as its budget, the number of people that can be used as team members on the project, as well as equipment and other resources that are available. All of these boundaries need to be accounted for in the planning process.

3.2 Resources

All projects require resources, even if it's just a few staff members and their time. Your project's success depends on making sure your team has considered all of the resources it needs before the project begins, and making sure the resources are available when they are needed. Large projects usually require many different kinds of resource. First, of course, projects need people. As mentioned, the project needs a manager, sponsor, and team members. Key stakeholders should also be identified. But there may be additional people who become involved in the project.

Next, your project may need other materials. These may include software applications and tools as well as actual materials that are part of the project. When planning the project, create a complete list of materials, the quantities you need of each, and how and when you will procure them. Remember any special equipment that is required. You may need computers, laptops, or tablets, or could require medical equipment and devices. If you are testing devices, you will want to select the models to test based on their benefits, drawbacks, and costs. Your project budget should include all of the costs the project will incur, including people's salaries as appropriate.[9]

3.3 Timeline

Developing an accurate timeline will go a long way toward ensuring a project's success. In the planning phase, the timeline can be one of the most crucial aspects of the project. Having subject matter experts on the team can help determine whether the timeline is realistic and achievable. Milestones you establish for each step of the plan may need to be adjusted.

The project manager determines how long each task will take, and then adds those together to find the total amount of time to reach project completion.

The work breakdown structure is a tool that fits its name: it breaks down the project into manageable sections. Each section has an associated deliverable, or product that indicates that section has been completed. The work breakdown structure is usually plotted in a flowchart. It can be thought of as an outline.

Consider project dependencies during the planning phase, as the timeline and schedule are created. Dependencies are simply parts of the project that must be implemented or resolved before other tasks can be completed. For example, data may have to be gathered, or surveys completed before the team can move forward. Understanding the dependencies helps the team put together a schedule that flows in a way that makes the most sense.[10]

3.4 Implementation

The plan is executed in the implementation phase of project management, beginning with the first step and following each step of the plan. Measuring the team's progress and monitoring any deviations needs to continue so that the plan can be updated as needed. Key deadlines and activities need to be communicated on an ongoing basis to keep all team members up to date. Make sure managers and stakeholders sign off on each completed task or step as required.

The project success plan is a specific communication planning tool the project manager can use to ensure that all team members and stakeholders understand what the plan needs to succeed. This is accomplished by meeting with the team and stakeholders early in the planning process and coming to an agreement on what defines project success. The project success plan should:

- Clarify all assumptions about the project and clear up any misunderstandings or disagreements
- Ensure all team members can work together and are efficient and productive
- Help keep the team focused and engaged[11]

3.5 Evaluation

After the project is complete, it is time to celebrate its successful conclusion. First, however, you need to determine whether it was in fact a success. The project should be evaluated by measuring its outcomes against its goals and objectives. The team should complete a post-implementation review that includes the following:

- Determine how closely the outcomes or results match the objectives. Are there any gaps?
- Review all of the project deliverables to determine their quality.
- Determine the satisfaction of stakeholders.
- Determine the project's costs and benefits.
- Identify areas for further development.
- Identify any lessons learned.

Methods for completing this post-implementation review and analysis include conducting surveys, distributing and collecting questionnaires, conducting focus groups, meeting with small groups and listening to feedback, and one-on-one interviews with key stakeholders.

All projects should be closed with a written report, usually written by the project manager with the support of the rest of the team. This report should assess the success of the project, catalog the project deliverables, note lessons learned, and officially end the project. It should include details for those reading it, such as the list of stakeholders, the project sponsor, and top leaders of the practice, to understand what the project accomplished and how it was completed.[12]

SAMPLE QUESTIONS

1. **What is the first step in initiating a project?**
   A. Define deliverables
   B. Define the practice's mission
   C. Define the scope of the project
   D. Determine costs

2. **Who determines how long each task in a project will take?**
   A. The project manager
   B. Subject matter experts
   C. Key stakeholders
   D. All project team members

Answers: 1-C, 2-A

TASK 4: SUPPLY CHAIN MANAGEMENT AND ASSET MANAGEMENT

Equipment purchasing and inventory control are key components in the operation of any medical practice. Medical groups must procure and distribute the right goods and services in the right place, at the right time, for the right price, and in the most efficient and effective way possible. Effective management of equipment and inventory requires competence in understanding the organizational objectives of the practice, knowing when to lease equipment and when to buy it, leveraging group purchasing options, and implementing an effective inventory control system.

KEY TERM

Group purchasing organizations (GPOs): Organizations that negotiate better pricing for the purchase of medical goods and services on behalf of their members.

4.1 Equipment Purchase vs. Lease Options

One of the many decisions your practice will need to make is when to buy equipment and when to lease it. There are many factors to consider when making this decision: capital availability, lease terms, how the equipment will be used, maintenance issues, why it is needed, and how do buying and leasing options compare?

Before any piece of equipment is acquired, the practice should analyze whether the new equipment helps to meet the organization's goals. The practice should examine how the equipment will be used, who will use it, and how it serves the intended purpose. Whether your practice has a purchasing manager, or other dedicated employee or committee for making these decisions, questions that should be asked could include:

- Will the equipment improve productivity?
- Will the equipment make the practice more successful?
- Will the equipment make the practice more competitive?
- Can the practice upgrade current equipment rather than acquiring new equipment?
- How soon will the equipment be obsolete or outdated?
- What are the maintenance considerations? (Will there be additional expense for a maintenance contract with a vendor, or will a staff member or clinician require additional training? Who provides the training?)

Also, remember that when purchasing equipment, the practice becomes the owner, while leased equipment is like renting, and the leasing company owns the equipment.

Figure 1.2

Pros of Buying	Cons of Buying	Pros of Leasing	Cons of Leasing
More affordable choice over the long term	Requires a sizable down payment	Little to no upfront costs	More expensive option for the long term
Increases the overall value of the practice	Equipment depreciation and obsolescence	Protects against outdated equipment	Monthly payments impact cash flow
Prevents the need for regular negotiations with the leasing company		Leasing companies may cover repair costs	
		Provides some tax benefits	

Two of the most important factors in equipment decision-making are capital availability and lease terms. The practice should consider whether it will need the capital for other purchases. If the capital needed to purchase new equipment is available and will not impact the practice's ability to fund other needed purchases, then purchasing the equipment or asset may be considered. Knowing the business's objectives for the year and in the coming years will help to answer this question.

Types of leases include:

A fair market value lease is one of the most common types of leases available. In this type of lease, the lessee is able to use the equipment for a specific period of time, usually 36-60 months. During this time, the lessee pays a fixed monthly fee for the use of the equipment.

A single payment lease is used when the lessee wants the benefits of leasing but has the capital available to pay the entire lease value up front.

A step lease is when the monthly payment amount increases or decreases over time. This might help a new practice as it grows.

Lease lines are similar to lines of credit. The practice is able to establish a maximum credit line it can use to lease additional pieces of equipment through the same vendor.

Early termination leases give lessees the ability to end the lease early. This is helpful if the practice believes a different piece of equipment may work better in the future.

Another important consideration is how the equipment will be used. Questions to consider include:

- Will it be an important part of daily operations or used occasionally?
- Will it be used for patient care or to support administrative functions?
- Will it improve efficiency or productivity, or is it required to meet regulations or safety codes?

Maintaining equipment, whether it is purchased or leased, is necessary for maximizing its value. Employees should be trained on its correct usage as well as how to keep it clean and operational. Some leases include maintenance agreements while others do not.

Other factors must be considered when determining if buying or leasing is best for the medical group. The purchasing or leasing decision should be made on a case-by-case basis to diversify the practice's range of assets. Also, the final decision of whether to acquire a capital asset and any leasing terms should be approved by the healthcare executive.

4.2 Group Purchasing Organizations

GPOs negotiate for the purchase of medical goods and services on behalf of their members, which include hospitals, nursing homes, medical practices, and other healthcare providers. Hospitals have used GPOs for several years, and increasing numbers of smaller medical practices are taking advantage of the buying power and economies of scale that GPOs can provide. Vaccines and medical supplies are often available through GPOs at discounts typically unavailable to smaller volume purchasers. By using GPOs, medical practices can sometimes avoid rising increases in costs of goods and supplies, or at least avoid a percentage of those increases.

GPOs also provide savings on administrative costs because they negotiate the prices with vetted vendors who are known to provide quality products on time. In addition, some GPOs have staff who can assist practices in developing and refining their purchasing process.

According to a 2017 report published by the Healthcare Supply Chain Association, GPOs can save provider organizations somewhere between 10 and 18% in purchasing expenses.[13] There are about 600 GPOs operating in the United States today. While GPOs provide many benefits, they are not free. The healthcare executive should ensure the practice has undertaken a thorough analysis of the benefits the GPO can provide and an estimate of the cost savings. Then, determine whether the benefits and cost savings outweigh the GPO's fees.

The GPO Safe Harbor was part of the 1987 Medicare and Medicaid Patient Protection Act and allows GPOs and vendors to form relationships that allow providers to realize cost savings on purchases without being considered kickback relationships. GPOs are still required, however, to meet all anti-kickback regulations.

4.3 Inventory Control Systems

Practices must also implement an inventory control plan to keep supplies organized, accessible, and easily counted. A good plan will also maximize storage space and track perishable items so they can be disposed of as they expire. Many practices have created par levels for exam rooms and the major supply closet, which determine proper levels of all supplies, from exam table paper to cotton swabs. Par levels normally will have three to four days' worth of supplies in each room and ensure that the supply closet has enough backup.

Label items properly to make navigating supply closets easy for those using and stocking items and to ensure that items stay organized. Move newer items behind older ones to rotate stock, and note expiration dates explicitly on perishables. For example, many vaccines are expensive and have short expiration dates, so using those with the shortest expiration date first will minimize waste.

Practices should consider wireless barcode scanning, which incorporates tablets into electronic supply management. Barcode scanning can also help to capture charges for items to be billed to insurance or the patient. Technology is also useful for automating supply chain management processes and can offer suggested orders based on history of use. It can reduce ordering time, maintain inventory minimum and maximum levels, streamline ordering processes, and track inventory and expiring products to reduce obsolescence and avoid excess inventory.

Unless properly controlled, the purchase, storage, and use of both billable and nonbillable supplies can become a significant drain on the financial status of the practice. Therefore, guidelines and operating procedures for the ordering, use, and monitoring of supplies should be initiated and maintained.

All employees who are involved in purchasing supplies should be trained in all aspects of the inventory control system. Training should occur with new hires and then refreshed at least once a year. Part of the training should emphasize the important role these employees play in the system.

Just-in-time ordering is another system that has become popular in the last few decades. It is an inventory system that notifies the purchasing agent when stock of an item has reached preset quantity. This quantity may represent the minimum quantity that the practice will need until an order is placed and received. The goal of this system is to ensure the organization has the materials it needs, but not more than it needs, and that restocking occurs in time before supplies run out. While this system may prevent overstock, there is also risk involved. Delivery disruptions such as unforeseen storms, for example, may cause problematic delays that can hurt the practice. Healthcare executives should monitor inventory and align supplies with patient trends, paying attention to seasonal needs.

The pricing component of the purchasing cycle is one of the biggest risk areas for fraud and irregularities. Practices must be careful about delegating purchasing authority to those employees who lack negotiating skills. Skilled, aggressive salespeople often woo these key decision-makers with small gratuities such as movie passes, sporting event tickets, meals, or gift cards to ensure their loyalty and convince them not to seek competitive bids or change vendors.

The control environment is an important consideration when evaluating a practice's purchasing cycle. A doctor or executive accepting gifts, gratuities, and other favors from medical suppliers, insurance agents, or major equipment vendors sets the wrong example for the practice's employees. Control is now heavily regulated through the Sunshine Act and should not factor into the practice's purchasing cycle.

A final category of supplies, which touches on all previous areas of discussion and has several additional issues, is pharmaceuticals. Within a practice, this category may have several distinct subgroups, based on the practice's specialty, including:

- Vaccines
- Injectable medications (e.g., Solu-Medrol, Depo-Medrol, vitamin B12)
- Narcotics
- Samples of prescription medications

The maintenance of pharmaceutical supplies within a practice is subject to various federal, state, and local regulations and laws. Narcotics and other controlled substances must be kept in secured locations (e.g., double-locked safes or metal boxes) that are not accessible to unauthorized staff members or others. Utilization logs for these drugs must be kept, and periodic inventories must be conducted. The logs for each pharmaceutical should document the final disposition of all narcotics and controlled substances purchased or received by the practice. All documents must be available to designated government investigators who have the responsibility to ensure compliance with regulatory safeguards.

The use of pharmaceutical samples within a practice poses significant issues regarding control, storage, and maintenance. Practices are swarmed by pharmaceutical sales representatives who provide information on why their particular pharmaceutical is the best and offer samples for patient use. The practice needs to implement inventory controls when accepting these samples to avoid accumulating significant excess quantities of specific drugs. Once the practice accepts samples for distribution to patients, it accepts responsibility for the proper storage, control, and ultimate disposal of the samples. In the event of a drug recall, the practice would need to ensure it can properly track who received a dispensed drug, so proper inventory control and reporting is critical.

Healthcare executives also need to consider the practical aspects of purchasing supplies. For example, the supply room needs to be large enough that optimal quantities of supplies can be stored there. The room needs to be organized so that supplies that are needed most often are the most accessible, and supplies should be rotated so that the oldest supplies are used first.

SAMPLE QUESTIONS

1. **A medical practice would choose a single payment term lease when it:**

   A. Expects to have more income over time

   B. Wants the benefit of leasing but has the funds to pay the cost of the lease in its entirety

   C. Wants to lease multiple pieces of equipment from the same vendor

   D. Wants to be able to end the lease early

2. **What is one advantage of a practice joining a GPO?**

   A. The practice is able to use a just-in-time inventory system

   B. The practice is able to obtain favorable leasing terms

   C. The practice is able to avoid rising increases in costs of goods and supplies

   D. The practice is able to avoid financing costs

Answers: 1-B, 2-C

TASK 5: FACILITY MANAGEMENT

The design, construction, maintenance, and appearance of a practice's office(s) are critical to the delivery of quality patient care as well as the efficiency of the practice. As with any business, the outward appearance of a facility establishes a foundation for patients' expectations of the level and quality of service they will receive. Key competencies required to effectively manage practice facilities include:

- Complying with general safety and life safety regulations
- Planning facilities for effective workflows
- Overseeing facility management and preventive maintenance
- Facilitating maintenance inspections
- Maintaining an environment of care, with appropriate protocols for infection control
- Managing proper disposal of biohazardous waste products
- Recognizing HIPAA implications

KEY TERMS

Gross lease: Property lease in which one monthly fee which covers all space expenses including utilities, property taxes, maintenance fees, etc.

Net lease: Property lease in which the tenant and the property owner divide the costs of the property.

Modified gross lease or modified net lease: Combination of a gross and net lease and is an option that many tenants and landlords find a good middle ground between the two.

Tenant improvement allowance: Agreement between tenant and landlord for payment of improvements to the property.

5.1 Maintenance, Safety, and Security

Employers realize how important occupational health and safety programs are to maintain a productive and highly efficient workforce. The cost of unsafe and unhealthy conditions in the workplace is substantial considering the lost productivity due to accidents and illness. In addition, the cost of providing workers' compensation coverage and healthcare benefits to employees continues to rise. The cost of providing safety and training programs is low when compared to the expense of employee accidents, injuries and illnesses, and workers' compensation claims.

More importantly, employees have a right to work in an environment that does not pose a health hazard or an unreasonable risk of injury.

The rise of worldwide disasters and the possible risks to healthcare workers and patients make such policies even more critical. Global pandemics such as COVID-19 also raise issues of exposure and risk to healthcare workers. Issues related to significant exposure to blood, bodily fluids, and tissues must be addressed, as well as exposure to contaminated needles, lancets, surgical instruments, incisions, and wounds. Another growing concern is exposure to hepatitis B and the need to administer the hepatitis B and influenza vaccines to those employees involved with direct patient care and supply handling. Musculoskeletal injuries are common in the healthcare industry.

Finally, employers have become aware of the importance of protecting the environment, community, and society in which they work.

Because of vandalism, pilferage, thefts, bomb scares, terrorism, and major incidences of workplace violence, securing your facility is important.

Security programs involve taking precautionary measures to ensure adequate protection of the group practice's property and assets, as well as the safety of its employees and patients. A group practice's security needs vary depending on its location, the nature of its operations, and number of employees. Some large groups hire security consultants to develop, administer, and audit their security programs, but even the smallest practice needs to create, implement, and enforce written security policies.

Managers should take terrorism seriously. The possibility of using everyday substances as biochemical weapons is a threat to both individuals and healthcare providers. Controlled substances should be kept in a secure place and monitored carefully, with only authorized individuals having access.

Before selecting any security system, the practice should perform a needs assessment to determine the level of security required. Factors that should be part of the assessment include:

- Location (security of the neighborhood, proximity to the police, fire station, etc.)
- Whether the practice is located in a freestanding building or inside a larger office building
- Whether the building is close to a busy street
- Size of the practice and if the practice accepts cash payments from patients
- Other considerations

5.2 Real Estate Management

If you are starting a new practice or relocating an established one, always keep your patients and staff members in mind when selecting a location. The optimal location is:

- In the approximate center of your market area
- Close to your primary hospital
- In a high-traffic, high-visibility area
- In a location with easy access to major feeder streets and highways

- With adequate parking that fits your patients' needs (easy access for wheelchairs walkers, pregnant patients, parents and caregivers transporting children, or patients with special needs, etc.)

Locating near your primary hospital may have the best combination of features, but may also have the highest cost, and the offices that are available may be unsuitable (e.g., have poor layout, difficult access, or inconvenient parking). Locating the practice near a hospital has drawbacks, especially if the hospital is a large medical center with numerous buildings and multiple parking lots in which patients may get lost. Keep in mind that the location requirements for a specialized practice may be different from family or general practitioners.

The best size for the office depends on a variety of factors. In the past, the general rule of thumb was to provide between 1,000 and 1,500 square feet of space per provider in the practice. While that can be a good starting point, determining the square footage is a much more complicated task today. Factors that play a role are:

- The type of practice (medicine or surgery)
- The number of practitioners
- Ancillaries (especially space-intensive areas for lab, X-ray, and bone densitometry facilities)
- Anticipated growth
- Support space (for records, staff breaks, etc.)
- A confidential area to discuss patient finances

Building or leasing an office demands careful planning for technical resources, especially network cabling, telephone cabling, and electrical outlets. Without careful planning, your office might not have enough outlets for computers or circuits might be overloaded during office hours, causing power disruptions. Installing cable after your office opens is expensive, time-consuming, and disruptive.

Do not sign a lease until the technology plan is set and you have reviewed it with the agent for the landlord. Be sure that the lease (or an addendum) specifies the party responsible for each component, as well as the right of the tenant group to change, add to, or alter technology features.

No matter how well a facility is designed and decorated, without proper preventive maintenance, the significant investment that is made in creating the facility will go to waste. Preventive maintenance includes such day-to-day issues as trash removal, vacuuming, dusting, and mopping. In addition, other maintenance items need to be scheduled on a regular basis, including window washing, touch-up painting, replacement of dim or burned-out bulbs, and minor cosmetic repairs of furniture and equipment. Mechanical, electrical, and plumbing elements should be inspected regularly to ensure that major problems are not imminent, so as to prevent hazards such as electrical fires and burst water pipes, which could have disastrous consequences. Make sure you understand who is taking responsibility for these items.

Paying attention to office design can prevent problems. Failure can result in problems that often compound one another. For example, an office layout that causes physicians and staff members excessive walking may lead to the duplication of expensive supply inventories within examination rooms to prevent fatigue.

When designing or renovating a facility, consider small details that enable a facility to be both efficient and attractive. Patients and visitors coming to the facility require appropriate signage to help them navigate from the time they enter the parking lot until they reach their destination within the building and then exit. Adequate signage is also important to assist new employees who are unfamiliar with the office and building layout. Appropriate color schemes for walls, flooring, and furniture are helpful in maintaining a relaxing and inviting environment for patients who might otherwise be stressed and anxious.

Many practices include quiet areas for older adults or separate play areas for children. Family medicine and pediatric offices often incorporate well versus sick child areas to minimize exposing healthy children to patients who are ill. As you will learn in an upcoming section, the design of the office should also account for people with disabilities. Guidance for patient access, such as requirements for ramps and elevators, are available at the ADA.gov website.

Competitive bidding is not often an effective tactic when negotiating leases, rent, and other costs related to the practice's real estate. Most practices cannot regularly move to a different location and are forced to negotiate with existing landlords or landlord brokers to get a better deal. As with supply negotiations, this often puts medical staff members in a position where they are engaging in something that is not in their skill set.

With an advocate, such as a tenant representative, practices can gain valuable assistance in the renegotiation and/or relocation of their practice to ensure that they get the best deal possible. Tenant representatives do not receive their compensation from the client. Instead, they receive a commission fee from the owner of a building in which their client elects to become a tenant. To ensure a smooth process, consider the options explained in the following sections when weighing real estate decisions.

Depending on the geographic area, the cost of financing a new medical practice is significant, and many banks have tightened their lending requirements because of the volatile economic environment. In addition, landlords require some type of security, such as a letter of credit from the individual practice owners, assuring personal liability to cover the costs of facility improvements.

Medical practitioners need to be prepared to cover relocation costs, which run from $150 to $250 a square foot, plus the cost of specialized medical equipment.

Office space can vary widely in cost from state to state, region to region, and from one neighborhood to another. Consider enlisting the services of a tenant broker or real estate attorney, or both, to ensure your practice is able to obtain the space it needs under the best terms possible.

A timeshare is another option for physicians and medical practices. In a timeshare, a facility has office space that is not being used and rents it for blocks of time, usually in four-hour increments, to another practice or physician. This often occurs when hospitals have built connecting office suites for patient examinations that are not being used.

Subleasing may also be an affordable option for medical practices. Subleasing occurs when a tenant no longer needs or wants a space prior to the end of the lease term agreement.

There are three main types of commercial leases. Healthcare executives should become familiar with each type of lease and consider the pros and cons of each before selecting one for their space.

The first type of lease is called a gross lease. In this type of lease, the tenant pays one monthly fee that can include utilities, property taxes, maintenance fees, etc. While the rent associated with a gross lease can be higher than others, it also becomes the only expense the practice has to pay. The advantage to this is that the rent stays the same even if utility costs and taxes increase.

Figure 1.3[14]

Type of Net Lease	Tenant Costs	Landlord Costs
Single net lease	Rent, portion of the property tax, utilities, garbage	Building expenses
Double net lease	Rent, portion of the property tax, portion of property insurance, utilities, garbage	Maintenance of common area
Triple net lease	Rent, portion of property taxes, insurance, common area maintenance	
Absolute triple net	Tenant pays all expenses for the property	

A modified gross lease or modified net lease is a combination of a gross lease and a net lease, and is an option that many tenants and landlords find a good compromise between the two. The modified gross lease gives both parties more ways to negotiate the lease terms.

Another factor to keep in mind is construction services, if improvements are needed before you can occupy the office space. You may work out improvement allowances, or TI allowances, with the landlord.

There are many factors that play a role in choosing to buy a property or lease one. Real estate can represent one of the practice's primary expenses, and this decision should not be made until a careful analysis has been conducted.

One pro of purchasing is that loan terms, such as the interest rate, may be more favorable for a practices because physicians typically have good credit histories, and they also stay in their property for many years. A purchase may make more sense when long term lease costs are expected to increase. If leasing costs increase while interest rates are low, or are expected not to rise dramatically, purchasing may be an attractive option. However, once a practice has purchased real estate and then brings in new providers who are not included in ownership of the building, it can present challenges, especially when existing providers are paying building costs.

The risks involved with purchasing are greater than those involved with leasing. Purchasing is a long-term commitment because selling the building and moving elsewhere can be a costly proposition. If the practice chooses to lease space, it is important to plan ahead for the end of the lease. Decide in advance whether to stay at that location or move. Be prepared to negotiate new terms each time the lease expires. Hire a real estate attorney or tenant broker to assist with the renegotiations. Also, track and understand when the landlord is required to notify the practice that the lease is nearing its expiration.

If the practice decides to purchase a building, practices are then responsible for all of the taxes, insurance, maintenance and other upkeep associated with the property.

If the practice is housed in a smaller, single-unit facility, managing it may be practical for the practice to do. However, if the practice purchased a multi-unit property leased to other tenants, it needs to perform a cost-benefit analysis to determine whether hiring an external management company would be beneficial. In some cases, hiring an external management company may provide cost or time savings to the practice.

The practice might also want to purchase a building in partnership with other practices or businesses. There are several different forms these partnerships can take. Real estate partnerships include:

- Joint tenancy: Two or more tenants own equal shares of the property
- Tenancy in common: Property is owned by two or more persons at the same time, but percentages of partnership vary
- Owning partnership: The property is owned by a limited liability company (LLC)
- Owning corporation: The property is owned by a corporation
- Owning trust: Property owned by a trust and managed by a trustee

The practice's attorney, and the partners' attorney should work with all parties involved to determine the type of partnership that would benefit the partners.

5.3 Compliance with Laws and Regulations

There are many rules and regulations imposed on practices. When the opportunity exists to design a new facilities plan, or to significantly renovate an existing space, it is best to use the expertise of an architect who is well-versed and experienced in the design and construction of medical office space. In designing or renovating facilities, applicable building codes and regulations must be integrated. These issues, which span local, state, and federal agencies, create a range of structural requirements that require compliance to ensure a safe environment.

Most facility-related federal regulations stem from the Americans with Disabilities Act of 1990 (ADA) and the Occupational Safety and Health Administration (OSHA).

The primary goal of the ADA, as it applies to facilities, is to ensure that individuals with disabilities have safe, easy access and can maneuver within a place of public accommodation. To comply with the ADA, building standards must address a host of physical design features. These include ensuring that doors are wide enough to allow for the passage of a wheelchair, providing restroom facilities that can be easily used by the people with disabilities, and providing adequate designated parking. In cases where the physical space is not owned by the practice, meeting these expectations is the responsibility of building management.

The safety of staff, patients, and visitors is addressed through adherence to the regulations set forth by the Occupational Safety and Health Administration (OSHA). These safety issues include the proper maintenance, use, and storage of equipment. They also apply to hazardous situations, such as loose extension cords, blocked hallways, and boxes that are stacked too high.

Properly identifying, collecting, and disposing of regulated medical waste (RMW) is a fact of life for a medical practice. OSHA strictly regulates and monitors the handling of hazardous medical waste, requiring proper labeling of hazardous waste containers, availability of those containers, and proper disposal of the waste contained in them. The rules surrounding RMW are complex and often imposed by several state agencies. Practices should consider streamlining RMW management by contracting with a reputable medical waste removal company that provides all of the containers your practice needs, disposes of the waste in them, and complies with all OSHA, state, and other regulations regarding that waste.

OSHA requires businesses to inform employees about hazardous chemicals, in compliance with the requirements collected in its hazardous communication standards (HCS) document. You can communicate the information through a comprehensive hazard communication program, which should include container labeling and other forms of warning, safety data sheets (SDS), and employee training.

The Occupational Safety and Health Act encourages states and territorial jurisdictions to develop and operate their own safety enforcement programs. These programs are approved and monitored by OSHA, which provides up to 50% of the operating costs. States must set safety standards that are at least as effective as the comparable federal standards. Typically, state-level programs adopt standards that are identical to OSHA, although states have the option to establish standards not addressed by federal rules.

The creation of an effective OSHA compliance program is a substantial responsibility for the healthcare executive. The complexity and diversity of OSHA standards are significant, and developing an effective program requires more than a cut-and-paste approach. Keys to success are:

- Organizational buy-in at all levels
- Employee involvement in identifying potential workplace hazards and solutions
- Training and documentation
- Constant review of the work environment and evolving OSHA standards

Facility management is a core part of a healthcare executive's job. The physical design and maintenance of the medical practice directly affects the quality of patient care and requires ongoing attention from the executive, with particular focus on safety as well as operational efficiency.

SAMPLE QUESTIONS

1. **A medical practice would use a joint tenancy real estate partnership when it is purchasing a facility:**

   A. In partnership with one or more additional practices and each owns an equal share

   B. As a limited liability company

   C. As a corporation

   D. As a trust

2. **OSHA considers proper handling of sharps a _______ consideration.**

   A. medical practice

   B. safety

   C. administrator

   D. physician

Answers: 1-A, 2-B

TASK 6: BUSINESS VENTURES

For many years, physicians operated their practices as sole proprietorships or partnerships and kept things as simple as possible. While this may have worked in years past, and may still be an appropriate choice for some, today's healthcare industry has become much more complex. Independent physicians are competing with hospital networks and medical corporations. Establishing a formal business structure and operation management system are important for practices to remain competitive and to reduce risk. When considering opening a new practice, practitioners should examine the types of business structures to determine which is best for the practice now, and in the future.

KEY TERMS

Business venture: A new business that forms based on a need in the market.

Independent physician association (IPA): Associations of independent medical group practices formed to contract with health maintenance organizations or for purchasing supplies or other services.

Limited liability company (LLC): One or more persons can own the company, but LLC separates the business from the owners so that personal assets may not be taken to pay business debts.

Sole proprietorship: Business owned by one person.

6.1 Types

The business venture forms and follows a definite plan with the expectation that it will earn a profit and the knowledge that there is also risk involved. Once the decision is made to open a new medical practice, the next decision is what type of business the practice will be. The primary types of business are:

- Sole proprietorship
- Limited liability company
- Partnerships
- Corporations
- Cooperatives[15]

The type of business structure selected will affect many things, including funding options, tax responsibility, and owner liability. Understanding the benefits, disadvantages, and potential legal repercussions of each type of business structure is important.

A sole proprietorship is considered the simplest business form available. One person is the owner of the business. That person is responsible for the decisions, funding, and legal obligations of that business. In this business structure, the owner of the company is not personally separated from the business. This is an important distinction as you will read about below. A sole proprietor is not a legal entity, but a person.

The biggest advantage of a sole proprietorship is control: The owner of the practice has control over the finances and all of the business decisions. In this business structure the owner does not have partners or shareholders to contribute to decisions. The owner has more flexibility when it comes to setting up and operating the business and making changes to those decisions as the need arises. It is also a simpler and easier business type to set up and manage.

There are several disadvantages of a sole proprietorship. They include:

- Lending issues: It is difficult for a new medical practice to borrow funds if it has no collateral. Most small practices may encounter this disadvantage. Borrowing often requires the physician to personally guarantee repayment of the loan.
- The owner assumes full liability, which means that the physician-owner, not a separate legal entity, is responsible for all liabilities (debts) of the medical practice.
- Full responsibility for all decisions is on the physician-owner. Some physicians may also view this as an advantage, rather than a disadvantage.
- The individual and business risks to the sole proprietor are greater than with other forms of ownership. This means that if the business fails, the owner's personal assets can be used to pay business debts. There may be some type of guarantee, but it will be limited.
- The owner pays employment taxes and does not receive a W-2; they must pay estimated taxes.

A limited liability company (LLC)[16] is similar to a sole proprietorship with some important exceptions. In an LLC, one or more persons can own the company. However, establishing the LLC separates the business from the owners so that personal assets may not be taken to pay business debts (unless the owners used personal financing to establish the business). Two specific types of LLCs that physicians may wish to consider are professional limited liability partnerships, or PLLPs, or professional limited liability corporations, or PLLCs. Both of these types of LLCs are specifically designed to structure businesses in which the owners are licensed professionals such as doctors or attorneys.

This structure protects the owners' personal assets. Another advantage is that there are fewer corporate formalities than in other corporate structures. Corporations must hold regular meetings of the board of directors and shareholders, keep written corporate minutes, and file annual reports with the state. The members and managers of an LLC are not required to hold regular meetings, which reduces complications and paperwork.

There are no ownership restrictions when it comes to LLCs. Other corporate structures like S corporations cannot have more than 100 stockholders, and each stockholder must be a resident or citizen of the United States. There are no such restrictions placed on an LLC. LLC owners also have the ability to deduct losses from their income tax returns. Members who are active participants in the business of an LLC are able to deduct its operating losses against the member's regular income to the extent permitted by law. Shareholders of an S corporation are also able to deduct operating losses, but shareholders of a C corporation are not. LLCs also provide their members with more tax flexibility than other corporate structures.

LLCs also present some distinct disadvantages that should be considered. For example, the practice's profits will be subject to Social Security and Medicare taxes. In some circumstances, owners of an LLC may end up paying more taxes than owners of a corporation. Salaries and profits of an LLC are subject to self-employment taxes. With a corporation, only salaries (and not the company's profits) are subject to such taxes. This disadvantage can be significant. A C corporation does not have to immediately distribute its profits to its shareholders as a dividend. This means that shareholders in a C corporation are not always taxed on the corporation's profits. Because an LLC is not subject to double-taxation, the profits of the LLC are automatically included in a member's income. LLCs also involve more complex governance, and it is more difficult to establish strong governance. Physicians are not considered employees. Physicians are generally not employees of PLLPs or PLLCs, so they usually are not entitled to the same benefits as found in a personal corporation or similar structure.

The primary types of partnerships are the general partnership, limited liability partnership, and limited partnership. In a general partnership, the partners will run the practice and assume responsibility legally and financially for it, such as assuming the debts of the partnership. A few examples of a general partnership include two partners opening a bakery, three partners opening an auto repair shop, or three partners opening a clothing boutique. In all of these examples, each partner is equally responsible for managing the business and ensuring its debts are paid. This also means that if one partner incurs business debt, the other partner is equally liable to pay it. Each partner needs to actively run the business.

Limited liability partnerships (LLP) work a bit differently. In this type of partnership, one partner is not liable for debts or legal costs the other partner incurs. One example of an LLP would be four attorneys who launch their own law firm. If one of the attorneys is involved in a lawsuit, the other three attorneys practicing with them are not liable to pay the costs of the suit. This may be attractive for physicians.

Figure 1.4[17]

Partnership Type	Advantages	Disadvantages
General Partnership	• No state filing is required • Few ongoing requirements • Two or more owners • Can be simpler to operate • Profits and losses attributed to each partner • Income allocated same as profit or losses, or can be different	• Unlimited business risk • Employment taxes need to be paid on all medical service income • Partnership must be dissolved if a partner leaves • Partners must pay estimated taxes (no W-2)
Limited liability partnership	• Personal assets cannot be used for business debts • Protects partners from one another's liabilities	• Partners must pay estimated taxes (no W-2) • Most expensive to create
Limited partnership	• Income can be distributed differently from ownership • Limited business risk for limited partners • Centralizes the management of the practice • Protects limited partner against business liabilities, but not from malpractice claims	• Employment taxes are paid on all medical service income • Partners must pay estimated taxes (no W-2)

Medical practices also have the option to form corporations. In a corporation, the owners hold shares in the company and so become shareholders. The four types of corporations available to medical practices are C corporation, personal service corporation, S corporation, and not-for-profit corporation. In a C corporation, the shareholders are taxed separately from the company. The company also needs to pay corporate income tax.

A personal service corporation is a specific type of C corporation. As the name implies, the business must provide a professional service, which is why physicians might choose to form one. The IRS rules for personal service corporations are that each employee-owner must provide at least 20% of the services and own at least 10% of outstanding stock in the corporation.

An S corporation meets specific IRS requirements. If the corporation has 100 or fewer shareholders or owners, it can be considered incorporated but is taxed as a partnership. This means that the company can pass income directly to the shareholders and not be taxed at the company level and the personal income level.

A not-for-profit corporation or nonprofit company, as its name implies, has a charitable purpose. All of its income must go toward running the business or achieving its goals. In other words, if a nonprofit's income exceeds its expenses, it is required to spend that money by investing it back into the organization or in other ways. By the end of the fiscal year, its accounting should show that income did not exceed expenses. In healthcare, this business type is most often used by hospitals, especially those associated with or created by religious organizations or educational institutions.

Some of the main advantages for practices forming corporations include the following:

- **C corporation**: Protects against personal liability for business claims, but not malpractice claims; can exist with no specified end and separately from owners; owner gets W-2.
- **S corporation**: Protects against personal liability for business claims, but not malpractice claims; can exist with no specified end and separately from owners; owner gets W-2; owners are taxed for profits and losses but shielded from business claims.
- **Limited liability**: Shareholders or owners are not liable for the debts of the medical practice.
- **Advantages of all types of corporations**: A key advantage of corporations is business continuity. Sole proprietorships and partnerships often dissolve when an owner or partner leaves. A corporation can continue when one of the partners leaves or retires. Corporations can receive extra tax deductions.

The biggest disadvantage to forming corporations is that the profits are taxable. Corporate-retained earnings are taxed, although this can be avoided in many instances by selecting S corporation treatment for tax purposes.

Corporations also must adhere to more complex governance limits control. The legal form of a corporation requires a governance structure with a board and elected officers. C corporations risk possible double taxation (on both personal income tax and business income tax). In an S corporation, income must be distributed according to ownership percentage and practitioners must have malpractice insurance. Both C and S corporations are more expensive to operate than other business types.

A less traditional business model that is gaining momentum is the healthcare cooperative, or co-op.[18] Medical or healthcare cooperatives provide an alternative model that allows physicians to have more control of the process, rather than insurance companies dictating so much of the process. In a healthcare cooperative, a group of general and specialty practitioners form a corporation that may be either for profit or not-for-profit. Facilities can include a wide range of diagnostic and testing equipment and services. Patients buy a membership to have access to the care options provided. Members are considered part owners of the company and the percentage of their ownership depends on the level of membership they purchase. Members have a vote in specific decisions related to the organization.

Memberships may be tiered so that patients can choose the level of care they believe is appropriate. Insurance is not required or used. The owner-physicians decide on the care and services needed for their patients. Some cooperatives include holistic services such as acupuncture and nutritional therapies.

The advantages to this model are clear: more physician control, a potential wider range of care options for patients, and flexible treatments. The disadvantages include a larger upfront challenge to begin a cooperative and raise capital. Members must also live up to their responsibilities for paying their membership fees, voting, etc.

In a joint venture, two already-established businesses decide to join forces for a specific reason that benefits both. For example, a medical practice would like to offer a specific diagnostic service and is located near a hospital that offers it. The practice and the hospital could embark on a joint venture agreement that would allow the practice to use the diagnostic services for their patients. The hospital benefits by bringing in more revenue. In a joint venture either business can decide to end the venture and still continue to do business.[19]

There is no one "right" choice when it comes to choosing the business type for a medical practice. The best choice will be determined by many factors, including:

- The potential risks and liabilities of your medical practice
- The costs and administrative requirements, and whether they are sustainable
- Any limitations on the number of owners
- The transferability needed
- Tax considerations to the owners
- Tax considerations to the entity

Also keep in mind that in some states medical practices are required to be set up as a professional or personal service entity. Check your state's requirements before selecting a business type. Also consider working with a business attorney to ensure you fully understand the business type you select, and to make sure the practice adheres to all laws and regulations.

6.2 Regulatory Issues

Medical practices must be aware of and comply with several laws:

Tax laws: How the business is taxed will depend on its business structure; in other words, whether it is a corporation, partnership, etc. There also may be property taxes payable if the practice owns property. In many states, sales taxes are not required to be collected or paid for personal service companies, such as medical and attorney practices. If any products are sold at the practice, sales tax will need to be collected. Medical practices should consult with a tax attorney to ensure they are compliant with all federal, state, and local tax laws.

Consumer protection laws: Consumer protection laws are enforced and overseen by the U.S. Bureau of Consumer Protection and the Federal Trade Commission. The goal of these laws is to ensure that businesses treat their customers fairly and according to the law. Medical practices are not exempt from these laws. Today, many of these laws relate to how consumer information is protected. Medical practices must comply with HIPAA and CMS regulations for protected health and personal information. Medical practices must also comply with specific rules about marketing and advertising.

Employment and labor laws: Medical practices must also be knowledgeable of and obey employment and labor laws that may describe how practices hire employees, comply with restricted work hours where applicable, offer required breaks, assure minimum wage requirements, etc.

Antitrust/fair competition laws: Antitrust and fair competition laws refer to the formation of ventures that could affect the ability of other companies to compete in the marketplace and limit the choices of consumers or patients. The goal is to provide fairness for others in the same type of business.

Interstate commerce laws: These laws refer to the sale of goods or services that cross state lines. If your medical practice expands to other states, the practice needs to be aware of and comply with these laws. Many acts over the years have defined interstate business practices, and the Federal Trade Commission oversees these practices.

License and permitting laws: Medical practices must ensure their practitioners at all levels are licensed to practice in their state. There may be other state and local licenses and permits that are required for practices to operate safely. For example, some local ordinances require elevators to be inspected on a regular basis and receive permits to operate. Fire inspections and certifications may also be required. Check state and local licensing and permitting laws to ensure your medical practice is meeting all requirements.

Contract laws: Contracts will be used in some employment situations, with vendors, suppliers, pharmaceutical companies, and in some cases, between doctor and patient. To ensure the contracts your medical practice writes, and signs, meet all legal requirements, have them reviewed by an attorney.

Intellectual property laws: Intellectual property laws refer to the rights patent, copyright, and trademark owners have to ensure their property is not being used without permission. Medical practices should be aware of these laws in order to understand what their rights are, as well as how to avoid violating any rules.

Financial regulation laws: Financial regulation laws refer to the laws governing financial transactions. These include credit card use, collecting on past due accounts, etc. See the *Financial Management* volume of the Body of Knowledge Review Series for more details about these regulations.

Bankruptcy laws: In the event that the practice must file for bankruptcy, there are laws and regulations at the state level that help determine how this is handled. There are different types of bankruptcy options. An attorney can help the practice through this situation. Practices may also need to be familiar with bankruptcy laws when collecting on accounts with patients who file for bankruptcy.

In addition to business types, medical practices have the option to join other partnerships and organizations that may benefit them. One result of the Affordable Care Act of 2010 was the formation of networks of physicians and hospitals for the purpose of coordinating care and to limit unnecessary or excessive spending. These organizations are called accountable care organizations, or ACOs.[20] ACOs are specifically designed for Medicare recipients. In order to qualify as an ACO, a network must serve a minimum of 5,000 Medicare patients for at least three years.

In order for ACOs to work, information must be available to all providers. ACOs benefit providers when they are able to keep their patients as healthy as possible. Doctors and hospitals must meet specific benchmarks provided by Medicare that focus on disease prevention and managing patients with chronic conditions. When the benchmarks are met, the network is paid a bonus by Medicare.

Independent provider associations (IPAs) and provider organizations (POs) are typically formed to organize independent medical group practices for the purpose of contracting with health maintenance organizations and purchasing supplies or other services. The main difference between IPAs and POs is that IPAs are typically affiliated with a hospital.[21]

The primary advantage of IPAs is that they offer a variety of physician choices to their members. They also tend to be more acceptable to managed care organizations (MCOs) than other, less traditional integrated delivery system models.

Because IPAs are one of the least-integrated forms of alliances, they do not offer the opportunity to leverage resources and achieve economies of scale that more integrated forms offer.

The term joint venture applies to a wide range of interorganizational arrangements and frequently refers to physician-related ventures. Joint ventures can provide medical practices with a competitive advantage, typically in an undeveloped or underdeveloped market, moving more directly from existing providers to a more convenient alternative for a targeted population. One advantage of joint ventures is that they can be quickly formed to take advantage of fast-moving opportunities. They also let organizations that are constrained by resources and capabilities pursue opportunities together by combining resources and expertise.[22] This can also lead to money savings for both entities.

Management services organizations (MSOs) are typically formed to provide management services and administrative systems to one or more medical practices. MSOs may conduct billing, marketing, and/or human resource functions for their members. Each medical practice remains a separate entity and chooses whether to use the services that the MSO offers. In addition to providing the preceding services, many MSOs purchase the assets of the physicians' practices.[23] MSOs allow small practices to leverage services they could not otherwise afford on their own.

There may be opportunities or reasons that medical practices seek to merge or to acquire other practices.[24] When two companies merge, they become one entity, which means redundancies are eliminated. Usually, mergers occur between two similarly sized businesses. It can make sense for two practices to merge if it will expand their respective markets and/or save costs. For example, a family practice with patients primarily on one side of town and a family practice serving the other side of town may want to merge to save costs. Mergers should be carefully considered.

Acquisitions usually occur when a larger company acquires a smaller one in order to gain a new market base or as a way to expand its market base or services. In some cases, a practice may seek to be acquired by another practice for similar reasons, such as expanding its market base or services, or gaining financial stability. For medical practices, much due diligence should go into the decision to acquire another practice.

Medical professionals must keep pace with rapid advances, manage complex reimbursement policies, understand technology, and comply with ever-changing government regulations. One way to meet these challenges, maintain and improve high-quality patient experiences, and maximize financial performance is to outsource nonclinical functions such as dictation/transcription, revenue cycle assistance, and miscellaneous office tasks.

Today's complex, automated practices have more options than ever when it comes to outsourcing, and more reason to leverage them. As your practice evolves, consider the following outsourcing options:

- EHR services help practices plan, select, and implement EHR applications.
- Financial planning services allow physicians to effectively protect their assets, maximize allowable income tax deductions, and design effective retirement plans.
- IT strategic planning can help healthcare executives understand the clinical, operational, financial, and technical aspects of IT planning and how it factors into the patient experience and bottom line. Typically, these IT professionals also offer core vendor planning and selection, systems integration, and security and disaster planning. IT management geared mostly toward healthcare organizations spans executive leadership, healthcare management, department administration, revenue cycle management, and IT management. Consultants can temporarily fill leadership roles.
- Remote and on-site systems management expertise, including system configuration, performance assessments, maintenance programs, and disaster recovery planning and implementation. Professionals can optimize overall IT investment, maximize system performance, minimize downtime, and reduce maintenance costs.
- Revenue cycle management can accelerate cash flow and optimize business office performance. Services can include interim billing management, revenue cycle assessment, coding and compliance management, performance metrics, and benchmarking.
- Web-based human resource management can automate tasks such as accruals, benefits, payroll management, and the Consolidated Omnibus Budget Reconciliation Act of 1985 (COBRA) administration. These services are often provided free or at reduced rates when the companies offer them as part of brokering insurance or other benefit programs.

SAMPLE QUESTIONS

1. Which is a requirement of a personal service C corporation?

A. The business must be owned by one individual

B. The business must provide a personal service

C. The business may not be owned by more than 100 stockholders

D. The business may not pass income directly to the shareholders

2. What is the purpose of an ACO?

A. To coordinate patient care and to limit unnecessary or excessive spending

B. To leverage services individual practices could not afford on their own

C. To provide management services and administrative systems to one or more medical practices

D. To provide training to all employees

Answers: 1-B, 2-A

TASK 7: INFORMATION TECHNOLOGY

Effective healthcare management is only possible when information technology (IT) provides useful information for good decision-making and assists in performing business and clinical processes; in other words, business intelligence (BI). Information management technology and BI are no longer adjunct, separate programs that support the practice. IT is a vital, integrated component that underlies ongoing success, especially when it comes to impact on quality care, closing service gaps, and patient information services. Key competencies required to effectively manage information systems include determining business needs and identifying goals; developing a technology plan, policies, and budget; selecting appropriate technological solutions; overseeing technology implementation; maintaining equipment; safeguarding information; and developing a technology disaster plan.

KEY TERMS

Database management system (DBMS): Converts large volumes of stored data into actionable information.

Electronic health records (EHRs): Patient records stored and transmitted electronically.

7.1 Evaluating and Selecting IT to Support Operations, Including Implementation Plans

The approach to assessing IT needs and then establishing a plan to address those needs is similar to the approach used in strategic planning. In fact, IT planning should be part of the overall strategy development process for the organization. This process includes evaluation of existing conditions and systems, consideration of alternatives relative to potential systems, selection of appropriate alternatives, and implementation.[25]

One of the best methods for identifying and addressing business process needs is to examine the practice's financial statements. Consider each line item as a potential opportunity for using technology to improve the bottom line.

Technology can certainly make your life easier. Electronic health records (EHRs) and practice management systems have been widely adopted, partly because they can be more efficient than handling reams of paper every day. However, as many vendors can attest, sometimes healthcare executives attempt to fix problems (such as scheduling or verifying insurance eligibility) with technology, even though adding a software program could make the process more complicated.

There are some key performance indicators that will help you determine whether your processes need to be streamlined. For example, you can benchmark your practice's performance indicators against better performers in the MGMA Performance and Practices of Successful Medical Groups to see how your practice compares. Some common metrics include percentage of total accounts receivable over 120 days and adjusted fee-for-service collection percentage.

You can also analyze:

- Claims denied at first pass, to pinpoint billing process pitfalls
- Percentage of copayments collected at time of service, to look at your front-desk reception performance
- Date of the third-next-available appointment, to identify patient access issues (Looking at the first-, second- and next-available appointments could be misleading because of last-minute cancellations.)

Any assessment should start with an inventory of all existing applications. The software may be integrated or may consist of several stand-alone systems. The final inventory prepared by an individual practice should include documentation on each particular software's standard capabilities, the age and costs of existing applications, and their strengths and weaknesses after the applications have been reviewed by the team. This information can be entered into a spreadsheet for convenient storage and access for analysis.

Business applications support the operational aspects of the practice, including scheduling, communications (including phone systems and all phone system applications), test and data management, and financial transactions. Common applications include:

- Practice management
- Services
- Claims processing
- Document processing
- Spreadsheets
- Databases
- Transcription
- Personnel management
- Inventory management
- Waste management
- Energy management

Clinical applications support patient care activities.

The drive for electronic health records (EHRs) originated with the need for easier handling and storage of documentation. Now EHRs are critical support tools for ensuring quality care and for enabling accurate billing for services.

When it comes to prescription management, newer prescription systems allow good documentation for care, guard against conflicting medications, and allow proper oversight for detecting misuse and abuse.

Good disease management programs allow the provider to assist the patient in proactive interventions rather than waiting until reactionary efforts are required.

They can reduce the overall costs of care for chronic diseases and improve the patient's quality of life.

Programs also need to address CMS's Merit-based Incentive Payment System (MIPS), in which physicians and hospitals receive financial awards from CMS when they meet specific care standards.

Patient applications are crucial for marketing and service delivery methods for medical practices. They include:

- Electronic communication
- Electronic monitoring
- Online education
- Telehealth

The importance of data security applies to all aspects of the software and hardware components of information management systems. A review of the systems with respect to the security of the information they contain, whether financial, clinical, demographic, or personal, should be made while inventorying the resources of the systems. The threefold approach established by HIPAA is an excellent method for reviewing the systems.[26]

The first review in the HIPAA approach should be the administrative systems, including the backup systems, disaster recovery systems, and emergency-mode operational capabilities. The second level of review should be physical resources. This includes hardware and software for workstations and storage media, as well as the overall physical facility. Finally, the technical aspects of the systems should be reviewed, including the authentication and transmission of data programs, data integrity systems, and other control systems.[27]

Steps for reviewing and analyzing the IT tech system include:

1. Conduct a risk analysis
2. Create a risk management strategy
3. Document your actions
4. Restrict usage outside the practice
5. Consider outside assistance
6. Establish contingency plans
7. Train and retrain staff

When performing an IT assessment, consider the needs of organizations and entities the practice interacts with, as well.

Regulatory agencies monitor activities and treatments more aggressively because policy interest is placed on the quality of outcomes, the costs of specific treatment programs, and disease management. The monitors search for better outcomes associated with a given approach and watch for abuses and misuses that may occur. Reference labs and diagnostic centers used by medical practices require clinical and financial information that practices typically collect. Shared information can yield cost and quality improvements for both the medical practice and the diagnostic service, but it is important to find ways to share this information in a confidential manner.

Inpatient programs need to know the treatments and drugs a medical practice provided to a patient prior to admission. The availability of current clinical information prevents duplication or omission of needed care and facilitates timely response to patient needs. The patient's financial information is also required to facilitate the reimbursement process.

One of the most difficult aspects of technology planning is predicting the future. Technology changes quickly and seldom in a linear fashion. Tremendous amounts of time can be expended attempting to monitor and assess the state of the art within the industry. Often this is an area for which the practice may wish to employ outside assistance. If the practice is considering growing or changing services, or becoming part of a larger or different organization, its future IT requirements may be dramatically different from those for the current clinical practice. For the healthcare executive, monitoring trends is a time-consuming but necessary requirement for determining the proper direction for the IT program. Outside assistance from an expert consultant may be valuable. Reliable IT vendors are a key source of information, not only about their own systems, but about industry trends as well. MGMA also offers seminars, books, and other materials that can help.

Although new information systems require less space than earlier systems because of their more compact design, the physical space requirements should still be considered. Proper ventilation, security, and utility support may dictate limits to hardware selections. Off-site or outsourced services may be required.

The lack of existing staff with the necessary IT support skills, or an inability to recruit such staff, may result in a decision to outsource IT services. A clear understanding of the system requirements for maintenance and upkeep should be made before selecting the equipment. If the practice staff is not capable of supporting the new systems, serious problems could result. The costs for providing long-term internal support versus the costs for outsourcing should be carefully compared.

Initial capital investment cost is often the least expensive component of an IT decision. Typically, the first year of operational support is built into the purchase agreement, but subsequent costs for upkeep may negate any initial benefits. Ongoing costs for staffing and consultation, support, updates, and hardware maintenance can overwhelm a medical practice, particularly a smaller one. Serious evaluation of the overall costs for the IT investment must be considered over an extended time. A five-year projection of costs and return on investment (ROI) will provide insight into the true value of the system.

Meaningful Use (MU) and the penalties associated with not complying with MU requirements should also factor into any IT infrastructure plan. There are often four main challenges associated with this:

1. Compliance. The vendor or product will not be able to meet government requirements for MU certification.
2. Usability. This often is a case where the technology seemed user-friendly during the vendor's demonstration but turned out to be anything

but once it was implemented, or once new demands were placed on it.

3. Customization. This involves buying an EHR that is purportedly ideal for a specialty practice — orthopedics, for example — only to discover that it needs to be customized based on each physician's specific needs.
4. Customer support. What kind of support are you able to get from the vendor? Sometimes this can be more specifically described as a lack of customer support.

The healthcare executive should consider several factors in planning the training process for a new system implementation or system upgrade. Business staff and clinical staff in the practice use different aspects of the information system's functionality, so training needs should be customized for each group.

Surveys are a good way to collect data about the staff's current knowledge and preferences for training programs. Based on staff size and the amount of information needed, the survey may be as formal as a written document to be completed and returned to the healthcare executive or as informal as an email with a few questions sent to all staff members.

The healthcare executive should determine the time required to complete training for all affected staff, being as realistic as possible. Creating a work schedule that maximizes staff productivity is a daunting challenge. Establishing a training schedule that doesn't adversely affect the work schedule can be difficult. Nevertheless, it is important that all staff members who are expected to use the information system receive training to use it correctly and efficiently.

The healthcare executive should establish a schedule that provides training first to staff members in key positions, that is, those individuals whose use of the information system is critical to business and clinical operations. Allow adequate time for key staff to master the required skills before training the next level of information system users. The schedule should also include makeup options. For example, if training occurs onsite during operating hours, the demands of the work environment may require staff members to abort training sessions to deal with pressing business or clinical matters.

Retraining needs should be considered as well. Few people can master difficult skills or change existing procedures in one session. It is usually a good plan to provide instruction, spend some time using the application, and return to the training mode to respond to questions or to verify that learning has been sufficient.

Today's healthcare workforce has access to more opportunities for professional development and continuing education than can be cataloged. High-quality programs are available on almost any topic of interest, and many programs are available in electronic formats that are accessible at the worker's convenience. The savvy healthcare executive determines what technology-based training solutions provide the greatest value to clinicians, to operating staff, and, in the long run, to the practice.

Available education resources are numerous, have a wide range of costs (financial, increased worker time), and are highly variable in their utility and quality. Managers planning for the education and professional development needs of the practice should draw from a variety of sources, but may rely primarily on a few tried-and-true sponsors. Representative categories of education sponsors include professional associations, proprietary organizations, and academic institutions. Perhaps most well-known to the healthcare executive is MGMA.

The healthcare executive should periodically review the professional development plan to adjust for changes in personnel or learning needs. The training budget should be monitored, and variances analyzed routinely with other budget elements. Most important, however, is the need to evaluate the actual learning outcomes achieved. The healthcare executive should meet with employees following training events and ask them to evaluate the experience based on a few key indicators, including:

- The instructor's expertise in the subject
- How well the program met the stated objectives
- The knowledge or skill gained as a return on time investment
- The knowledge or skill gained as a return on financial investment

Over time, patterns of responses may emerge that affect the healthcare executive's future selection of education vendors and choices for approaches to training.

7.2 Data Capture, Aggregation, and Analytics

The ultimate purpose of a database management system (DBMS) is to convert large volumes of stored data into actionable information. Medical practice management is full of changes and shifting priorities, so the value of an information management system is tied to the ease with which information can be accessed, manipulated, securely shared, and presented to support decision-making.

Most medical practice data, such as patient records, treatment reports, accounting data, schedules, and appointments, are held in some form of database. Some data sets are in relatively simple "flat files," such as spreadsheets, that are easily updated and manipulated and require minimal management. Other databases, such as relational databases, comprising multiple tables of data, require more active management.

As with most aspects of management, the first step in planning DBMS development is to conduct a needs assessment. A DBMS in a practice allows management of data to help drive business decisions. Databases allow definition of data types and data formats for the stored information. Each variable in a database is contained in a field. An example of a field is a patient's last name.

Databases store information in a record. A record is a collection of multiple related data fields, perhaps about a particular patient or inventory item. For example, the fields comprising a patient's complete demographic information or clinical data from an encounter are stored as a record. In the database, records are displayed in an electronic form, where field data may be entered, edited, viewed, and deleted. Several records with the same related fields of information for entries are referred to as a database table. The data contained in database tables can be presented in a formatted, easy-to-read report. A single report could contain data from many different tables and incorporate a complex set of relationships created by using multiple links within the database.

The DBMS administrator should work with key clinical and administrative staff to develop policies and procedures ensuring the security and confidentiality of the practice's identifiable health data.

At a minimum, plans, policies, and procedures should be established for the following DBMS issues:

- Regular, routine data backup
- Journal or log for documenting alterations to operational software
- Formal process for database maintenance by authorized personnel
- Physical database security
- User access control and monitoring
- Database recovery plan

The medical practice must ensure that its electronic network and information systems are secure. Any security program in a healthcare organization should have three principal goals:

1. Protecting the private information of patient-related data
2. Ensuring the integrity of information
3. Ensuring the availability of information to the appropriate individuals in a timely manner

Employers may need to be identified when they transmit information to health plans to enroll or disenroll an employee as a participant. Whenever information about the employer is transmitted electronically, it is beneficial to identify the employer by using a standard identifier.

On May 31, 2002, HHS published the Final Rule for Standard Unique Employer Identifiers, which required that the Internal Revenue Service Employer Identification Number be used as the standard identifier of employers in HIPAA-covered transactions.[28]

The HIPAA Privacy Rule established standards for who may have access to personal health information (PHI) and how the information can be used. Key provisions of these standards include:

- Patients' access to their medical records
- Notification to patients of their providers' privacy practices
- Limits on how providers may use personal medical information
- Restrictions and limits on the use of patient information for marketing purposes
- Assurance that providers take reasonable steps to make their communications with patients confidential

The HIPAA Security Rule sets the standards for ensuring that only those who should have access to ePHI have access to it. The rule requires a three-pronged strategy: (1) technical safeguards, (2) administrative safeguards, and (3) physical safeguards. Technical safeguards include access controls, audit controls, data integrity controls, authentication, and transmission security. Administrative safeguards include backup plans, disaster recovery plans, an emergency-mode operation plan, and testing and revision procedures. Physical safeguards include facility security, device and media control, and workstation use and security.

HIPAA identifies data confidentiality, integrity, availability, and accountability as the primary areas of concern. Access controls are measures to ensure that only authorized personnel have access to a computer or network, or to certain applications or data.

A major purpose of the HIPAA Privacy Rule is to define and limit the circumstances in which an individual's PHI may be used or disclosed. As a rule, the medical practice may not use or disclose PHI except as the Privacy Rule permits or requires, or as authorized in writing by the individual who is the subject of the information, or authorized by the individual's personal representative, such as a parent in the case of a minor.

The medical practice must develop and implement policies and procedures for releasing PHI. Procedures must also be established to document the process of restricting access and use of PHI based on employees' specific job roles. These policies and procedures must identify the individuals who need access to PHI to conduct their duties, the categories of PHI to which access is needed, and any conditions under which they need the information to do their jobs. These policies and procedures should reference state regulations and other federal regulations that govern the disclosure of protected patient information, such as the Confidentiality of Alcohol and Drug Abuse, Patient Records Regulation, the Medicare Conditions of Participation, and the Clinical Laboratory Improvement Amendments, if applicable.

System integrity is grounded in protecting the information system and the data it contains against tampering. Unauthorized access is one of the most serious threats to security in any information system.

Prevention of unauthorized access relies on a good access control system. Passwords and user identification have been discussed previously as the primary mechanisms for controlling access to the information system and its data by practice staff.

Recommendations for content in the confidentiality statement include specifying that practice staff will:

- Not use practice email for personal messages
- Never open or redistribute attached files from an unknown source
- Never send confidential patient information in an email unless it is encrypted
- Always verify the address line of an email before it is sent
- Never share passwords

- Never log in to the information system with someone else's password
- Always keep computer screens pointed away from public view
- Never remove computer equipment, disks, or other portable storage devices, such as jump drives or software, from the facility without the express permission of the healthcare executive

Consequences for breaching privacy and ignoring security practices should be explicitly stated and communicated to all staff. Consequences established by the practice should be determined by the severity of the infraction and may range from written warnings to immediate termination. Put these policies in writing, distribute them to all employees, and incorporate them into your training (documenting that you did so).

The failure of data storage systems is not a question of if, but when. As medical practices increasingly adopt EHRs, their leaders must not overlook the protection of valuable data.

Evaluate business recovery plans that include the recovery time objective (RTO) and recovery point objective (RPO). RTO is the acceptable or contracted downtime for a computer system. The cost of EHR systems varies greatly. While some systems may only cost a few hundred dollars per full-time equivalent (FTE) physician, they deliver little more than a medical word processing program compared to full-featured, robust, and integrated front and back-office systems that cost thousands of dollars per FTE physician.

Even these costs vary, depending on whether new hardware is required and how software is deployed (as a stand-alone system or licensed as an online application). Equally important is RPO, the amount of data that can be lost. Essentially, RPO represents the time between the last data backup and a disaster. When setting the backup frequency, physicians and staff members should consider how far back they could remember if they were forced to recreate an EMR. Specialists who see few patients in a day, for example, can make backups less frequently than a specialist who sees dozens of patients a day. Ideally, healthcare executives determine balance between RTO and RPO. Systems that offer short RTOs and minimal RPOs (including those that support continual backup) are available, but they cost more.

Several options for protecting and recovering data are:

Tape backup: External or internal tape drives and magnetic tapes store duplicate disk files. Removable disk drives accomplish the same task. You remove the old tape or drive and install a new one daily.

Image capture: Although more expensive than tapes, this option can have an effective RPO because images are captured more frequently. Like physical tape storage, image archives should be maintained off-site for disaster recovery.

Outsourcing: If your group is small and has few internal IT resources, consider outsourcing data backup and recovery. Vendors usually conduct backups on a guaranteed schedule that does not interfere with practice operations, and recovery times can be customized.

Application Service Provider (ASP): Many EHR providers offer their products under this model, which allows practices to license the use of the EHR but not install software on their local servers. Instead, professionals install a small "client" program on local computers.

Computers play a crucial role in medical practice operations. That role will only grow with the expansion of EHR systems, which heighten the importance of data security and integrity. To get the right protection, here are a few suggestions:

- Hold frank discussions with physician users to determine comfort levels with system downtime (RTO), as well as how much data loss is tolerable
- Learn how much physician users are willing to pay for data security
- Decide whether to keep data recovery in-house or contract with a service
- Write a plan for disaster prevention and recovery, and test it annually

Cloud-based technology is becoming a more readily available option for practices deciding where to store their patients' health information. Cloud storage involves storing data (patient, clinical, and financial data in the case of medical practices) in a virtual storage pool, which is typically hosted by a vendor.

Cloud-based systems can be cheaper than stand-alone software programs. Many cloud-based vendors offer subscription fees to the service, usually on a monthly basis. Paying the fee allows the practice to access the records with a computer and internet connection; no other hardware or servers are needed. Unlike a standard equipment purchase or lease, the upfront cost is very low.

With cloud-based storage there is no downtime from systems having to upload applications and interfaces. Cloud-based systems usually update and back up automatically. This means every user in your practice will have the same software version and will be working with the same information and data.

Cloud-based storage plans often offer less expensive disaster recovery solutions compared to other options. If the practice has a fast internet connection, it can download data from the cloud, and most plans support versioning so you can revert to an earlier version of a file if the newer one becomes corrupted.

Aggregated data, as the term indicates, is patient data that is collected and analyzed together as a whole, such as what were the diagnoses of all patients treated at the medical practice, what are the ages of patients at the practice, etc.

Data can be aggregated to capture counts during a specific timeframe, to track patient data for specific providers, organizations, and patient populations. Data can and has been shared across many practices and providers for the benefit of learning more about specific diseases and treatments. There are repositories of data that can also be accessed. It is important to keep in mind that in some circumstances you must get patient permission before sharing data with those outside your medical practice.

Data aggregation and analytics are used commonly for the following reasons:

- Finding opportunities for improvement/quality improvement
- Reporting public health concerns
- Improving patient outcomes

- Finding common characteristics that might predict the course of a disease
- Monitoring healthcare trends
- Providing research/education
- Facilitating better healthcare products
- Streamlining or reducing patient care costs
- Maintaining transparency and trust
- Finding new marketing opportunities

Leveraging the power of technology is a cornerstone of effective medical practice management. Key skills in this area include identifying technological opportunities tied to business goals, obtaining and implementing particular technology systems, safeguarding the integrity of systems and data, and mitigating risk to technology in the event of disaster.

SAMPLE QUESTIONS

1. **Which is a critical IT process related to patient care?**
   A. Claims denied at first pass
   B. Transcription
   C. Personnel management
   D. Online education

2. **What is one advantage of cloud-based storage systems?**
   A. They are the same cost as other storage systems
   B. They offer disaster recovery systems that are the same cost as others
   C. They update and back up data automatically
   D. They offer longer downtime for loading

Answers: 1-D, 2-C

TASK 8: COMMUNICATIONS, MARKETING, AND COMMUNITY RELATIONS PLANS

Marketing for a medical practice involves activities associated with identifying patient needs and satisfying those needs. Typical marketing tasks may include market research, patient needs analysis, strategic decision-making about service design, and promotion of the practice. These marketing tasks can be best accomplished when analyzed through the four A's of marketing for medical practices: access, availability, accountability, and accommodation.[29] Keeping patients at the forefront of your marketing plan will ensure that a practice's services best match patients' needs and expectations.

Key competencies aligned with effective marketing management in a medical practice include: understanding the local market and community resources, developing a marketing plan, applying aspects of the plan to establish a corporate image, understanding digital marketing, using social media and reputation management wisely, using public relations to promote the practice, and collaborating with community organizations to foster patient health.

KEY TERM

Search engine optimization (SEO): Long-term strategy focused on improving overall visibility of a site in search engine results.

8.1 Local Market Environment

A marketing plan is similar to the strategic plan discussed in Task 2 and needs to be developed using the following framework:

- Executive summary
- Situation analysis
- Market research
- Market strategy

The executive summary of the practice's marketing plan should address the following key elements:

- What are the dominant issues discovered in the practice's situation (SWOT) analysis?
- What are the key objectives — in the shortest possible form — the practice seeks to achieve?
- What, in one or two sentences, is the practice's marketing strategy to achieve those objectives?
- What other concepts unique to the practice should be addressed?

Answers to these questions comprise the body of the marketing plan; therefore, the executive summary cannot be written until the plan has been completed. It will then serve as the "snapshot" of what the practice aims to accomplish with its strategic marketing.

The situation analysis investigates the macro- and microenvironment in a manner similar to the strategic plan. In fact, the strengths, weaknesses, opportunities, and threats (SWOT) analysis discussed earlier in this book can be used in this stage of the marketing plan process. The practice should review its strategic plan's SWOT and then consider each of the SWOT's components from a consumer and market viewpoint, including external threats and opportunities, internal strengths and weaknesses, key success factors in the healthcare industry, and the practice's sustainable competitive advantage.

Macro-environmental analysis refers to continuous structured data collection and processing on a broad range of environmental factors, such as the economy, competitors, payor activity, the governmental and legal environments, technology, and social culture. This allows the practice to act quickly, take advantage of opportunities before competitors do, and respond to environmental threats before significant damage is done.

The microenvironmental, or internal, analysis seeks to uncover the resources of the practice that apply or can be applied to marketing efforts. These resources include money, time, people, and skills. The key question to ask is what internal resources does the practice have that are underexploited? Finding these resources internally as opposed to having to seek them externally provides countless benefits to the practice. Along with identification of resources, the practice's vision, mission, and goals (in particular, long-term goals and objectives, marketing goals and objectives, and financial goals and objectives) should be reviewed, and the culture of the practice should be considered. Each of these areas has an influence on the marketing strategy of the practice. Also, it's important to note that an internal analysis today should include reputation management and a review of online comments.

A consumer analysis explores the demographic makeup of the practice's consumer base, but also delves a bit deeper into the consumers' purchasing and decision-making behaviors, their motivations and expectations, and loyalty segments.

The final piece of the situational analysis is the market analysis. Here the medical practice defines its market; identifies its market size and industry market trends; evaluates the market segmentation and strategic groups; and studies the competition's strengths, weaknesses, and market share.

Marketing research is the next major task in the marketing planning process. The American Marketing Association defines it as: "...the function that links the consumer, customer, and public to the marketer through information used to identify and define marketing opportunities and problems; generate, refine, and evaluate marketing actions; monitor marketing performance; and improve understanding of marketing as a process. Market research specifies the information required to address these issues, designs the method for collecting information, manages and implements the data collection process, analyzes the results, and communicates the findings and their implications."[30]

The aim of marketing research is to answer the following questions:

- Who are the customers?
- What services do they want?
- When do they want these services provided?
- Where do they want these services provided?

Answers to these questions can reveal problems with current services and potential trends for the future. Market research should also help the practice determine its market share and the effectiveness of its advertising and promotions.

Three general sources of market data can be gathered:

1. Data already available externally (e.g., from chambers of commerce, business coalitions, state trade organizations, and the U.S. Census Bureau)
2. Data readily available internally (e.g., from employees, current patients, and company records and files)
3. Data that can be collected by and/or for the practice (e.g., through surveys, interviews, evaluation and response cards, customer feedback, and observations of competition)

If you have been practicing in the area or have been a resident nearby, you should have a good idea of several key indicators:

- Patient volume
- Underserved needs
- Insurance contract availability
- Percentage of patients with Medicaid or Medicare
- Percentage of uninsured patients
- General economic climate
- Business and industrial base (including the major health insurers)
- Supply of physicians in your specialty, including:
  - Physicians approaching retirement
  - Physicians recently recruited to the area
  - Physicians within driving distance for your patients
  - Specialty centers whose physicians could compete with you

Other marketing tips to keep in mind:

- Constantly appraise your patient population
- Know what the community wants
- Know your competition
- Census-tract data can show high-demand areas
- Obtain market data for your region
- The strategic plan should guide expansion
- The strategic plan and market awareness should guide change

After the market research is completed, the next step is to develop a market strategy describing the broad plan to achieve the practice's marketing goals and objectives. This may include using the information and data collected to determine consumer wants and needs that are not being met by the practice or by the competition, or determining areas where new services or different services would capture new markets.[31]

To develop a marketing strategy, the practice needs to identify a target market. This is a specific group of consumers who have a want or need for the practice's services or products.

Market segmentation — the method of grouping a market into smaller subgroups — is the process of target marketing. Market segments can be geographic (certain regions or climates), demographic (age or race), psychographic (attitudes, behaviors, lifestyles, or loyalty characteristics), or historical (previous customers). If the practice's services are confined to a specific geographic area, then the target market can be further defined to reflect the number of users of the service within that geographic segment.

Once target markets are identified, the practice needs to develop a marketing mix that is positioned to be attractive to that segment. The marketing mix enables practices to join together different marketing decision areas, such as products, prices, promotions, and place (also known as E. Jerome McCarthy's 4P's) to develop an overall marketing plan.[32]

Products: In medical group practices, products are typically services. In determining the marketing mix and developing the marketing plan, these services should be used as marketing resources, and a focal point should be differentiation of the practice's services from those of the competition.

Prices: Determining and setting prices for a medical practice and the visits or procedures that are offered is not a simple process. It is important to look at insurance contracts, the amount allowed, and if there are procedures or visits that are not covered under insurance that need to have cash or self-pay prices set.

Promotion: Communicating with and selling to potential customers requires promotion, including sales promotions, advertising, and public relations (only the latter two are applicable to most group practices).

Place: Place, meaning placement or distribution, refers to decisions regarding market coverage, member selection, logistics, levels of service, and convenience to the customer.

Positioning: Although not a part of McCarthy's original 4Ps of the marketing mix, there is a fifth P — positioning — for practices to consider as well. This is the special niche your practice occupies in a customer's mind. A practice's positioning strategy is affected by a number of variables that are closely tied to the motivations and requirements of target customers as well as the actions of primary competitors.

The culture of the practice, in contrast, is informal, flexible, created and maintained by word of mouth, and ideology centered. It defines good and bad, winning and losing, friends and enemies, and so forth.[33] The cultural characterizations of the practice — people, circumstances, events, objects, facts, processes, and information — are critical for practice decisions and progress.

Structure and culture are unique to each practice and shape the image that the practice presents to the community.

The final component of the marketing plan is advertising, which, as mentioned earlier, relates to promotion. Gone are the days when a practice could "hang out a shingle" and the phone would begin to ring. Healthcare is an extremely competitive marketplace that requires practices to engage in innovative advertising practices.

The choice of advertising method should be guided by the answers to the following questions:

- What is the source of the practice's current patients?
- What method is optimal for conveying the practice's "message"?
- What method will reach the largest concentration of potential customers?
- What is the cost per unit (i.e., new patient) for this type of method? What is the expected return on investment (ROI)? The cost of the acquisition of a new patient compared to the revenue a new patient brings in may be appropriate, but applies to specific services of the practice as well.
- Is this method ethical in all possible respects?

Once an advertising method has been selected, the practice needs to ensure that the materials designed are written at an appropriate reading level and are clear, concise, and appealing, and take into consideration the population most likely to be served by the practice. Advertising materials, as with all other components of the marketing plan, also need to portray the practice accurately and honestly.

8.2 Referral Analysis

Referrals continue to be an important source of obtaining patients for most physicians, especially those that specialize. A GP's office may get more results from aiming marketing at consumers, but specialists depend on referrals as a source of patients. Healthcare executives should have a detailed idea of where the practice's referrals are coming from and perform an analysis on these sources to identify where there may be opportunities to improve the flow of referrals from particular sources, or to identify when an important referral source begins to decrease its referrals.

Today, there are laws and regulations that practices must comply with when it comes to referrals and how to gain them. The Anti-Kickback Statute (AKS) and Stark laws have been discussed in other chapters of this volume. However, they need to be viewed through the lens of referrals here.

Violating the AKS can result in both criminal and civil penalties. It regulates how providers can market to referral sources. In the past, some practices provided gifts and entertainment to referral sources. The AKS strictly prohibits gifts and entertainment when used as a way to reward referrals. Dining with a source is considered OK as long as the purpose is to discuss business details and not as a reward or incentive for continued referrals. Cash incentives for referrals are never appropriate.

Stark laws were enacted to prevent physicians from referring patients to other practices or facilities in which they have economic ownership. For example, it is against the Stark Law for a physician to refer patients to an imaging center that the physician owns, in part or whole. This also includes referring patients to other practices or providers who are family members of the practice. When designing a referral plan, the healthcare executive needs to ensure it complies with these laws. The practice may want to have an attorney who specializes in healthcare law review the referral plan before it is executed.

There are a number of ways practices can market to referral sources that comply with marketing legislation. The important thing to note is that the practice needs to develop a referral source marketing plan and stick to it. Here are some ideas to consider for the plan:

- Be visible in the medical community by attending health fairs, conferences, and local medical association meetings
- Communicate with referral sources regularly
- Welcome new providers
- Meet with current providers
- Advertise
- Evaluate referral sources and update them regularly

Keeping track of the referrals the practice receives is integral to managing the marketing plan, especially when referrals are a major source of new patients. If your practice isn't already tracking referrals, start by analyzing where they are currently coming from. List all referrals by provider, and determine how many patients are being referred from each provider, and how often. If your practice offers a broad range of patient services, also list which services were referred.

Once you have a good understanding of where your referrals are coming from, you can begin to develop a plan for maximizing the referrals you're currently receiving and target new providers. Make sure tracking includes internal as well as external sources.

Referral tracking should continue and be analyzed on a monthly basis, as well as yearly. For example, if during the same month the previous year referrals from a few sources were much higher, that may be a signal to find out why they are lower this year. Or if referrals vary greatly from month to month, it is important to understand if they are related to a natural seasonal variance, or whether the sources have turned to other practices to refer patients. Decide what key performance indicators (KPIs) and benchmarks are important for your practice to use in its analysis. You might also consider using referral source tracking software that will automatically produce reports according to the KPIs and benchmarks you've chosen.

8.3 Legislative Awareness and Advocacy

In addition to the Anti-Kickback Statute and Stark laws, medical practices must comply with the Centers for Medicare & Medicaid (CMS) marketing regulations. CMS has published a 120-page document that outlines all of its guidelines and regulations when it comes to marketing. Practices should take the time to understand all of these guidelines. The most important to note are:

- All advertising or marketing claims must be true
- Guidelines for when and how to call patients must be observed
- There are limits on when the practice may advertise or market new services or physicians who are new to the practice
- Patient information must be protected

Today's healthcare executives should also be willing to become legislative advocates by developing relationships with federal and local representatives. Doing so benefits the representatives by giving them a deeper understanding of the healthcare industry and concerns associated with it, and executives can communicate those concerns and advocate for legislation that addresses the practice. Healthcare executives should meet with local and federal representatives as well as join or participate in any advocacy groups organized by local and national medical associations.

While there are no specific laws or guidelines specifying whether physicians can receive gifts, including payments, from patients, the American Medical Association discusses the ethical reasons behind when to accept and not accept patient gifts.

When patient gifts are offered in gratitude to the physician and do not represent a financial hardship to the patient, they are acceptable. There must also be clear understanding that the patient is not expecting preferential treatment of any kind if the physician accepts the gift.

Patient gifts that seem to be extreme or out of proportion to the sentiment expressed, those that appear to be a request for preferential treatment or to influence medical care choices should not be accepted by the physician.

8.4 Marketing Strategy

Medical practices should consider the pros and cons of the many promotional and advertising channels open to them. These include, but are not limited to:

- Digital advertising, including pay-per-click advertising
- Print advertising
- Broadcast advertising, radio and television
- Face-to-face channels
- Mobile channels

The pros and cons will vary according to the type of practice and the practice's marketing goals.

Although many large healthcare organizations and health systems are using the power of social media to engage patients, social media experts say smaller private physician groups and individual physician offices are only cautiously dipping their toes in the social media pool. Healthcare professionals may be reluctant to interact with and engage patients online, given potential HIPAA privacy issues and other challenges. However, with a carefully crafted social media policy governing the use of networking tools for the organization — and an appropriately executed strategy — many organizations are realizing the benefits of social media. Your practice can reach out to inform, educate, build rapport, and increase patient trust through open, real-time communication with patients.

When using social media, develop a clear and concise plan for online activity. Identify the practice's goals, audience, and where those patients connect online. Here are some additional questions to ask:

- What resources does the practice have to allocate to this new marketing initiative?
- Who will manage this strategy once it has been developed?
- What legal implications must be considered as the practice moves forward to protect patient privacy?

Managing various social media channels is more time-consuming than you think. Social media's power lies in its immediate nature and back-and-forth dialogue, especially platforms such as Facebook and Twitter, so be ready to respond to patient complaints and compliments quickly.

Social media sites can be used to communicate with patients about everything from weather or holiday closings to special events and center donations. They can be a place to share staff birthdays, information about new clinics, and biographies of new physicians and staff members. Used to its full potential, social media lets the practice create a dialogue with patients about important or even lighthearted topics.

Although the cost of using social media is minimal, it takes time to build and cultivate a social media presence. It's essential to develop a robust profile on whatever social media channel the practice chooses to focus on. It's not enough to just throw the practice's name up on a social media site. Invest some time to create a dynamic presence, which might include staff photos and biographies, a virtual tour of your office, and updated contact information. Imagine that this is the first place a patient learns about the practice. Put the practice's best foot forward and spend time making the profile reflect the work the practice does to serve patients.

Once the website and social media avenues are up and running, continue to devote time to posting and monitoring the social media accounts. It's recommended that someone on the staff be designated to devote about a half-hour a day to share new information and engage with practice followers. Assign a few employees to post on the practice's behalf and ensure that they are professionally trained and can represent the practice's "voice" effectively and responsibly.

Remember to be creative. Develop special promotions, share exclusive information, or run a practice referral contest on the chosen social media platform.

Don't be afraid to think outside the box and brainstorm new ways to interact with the practice's fans.

The goal of a practice's social media is to provide relevant, local, and engaging content to showcase how the practice is connected to our communities. Facebook is a good primary focus, as it is the top channel for many practices' target audience.

Goals for Facebook:

- To serve as an additional platform for users to find and interact with a clinic and its brand
- To maintain a consistent, accurate brand presence
- To serve up timely, helpful content to a practice's followers
- To acquire and respond to reviews on our location pages
- To connect with our local communities

How does a practice determine its paid media spend?

- Evaluate each channel for the most efficient cost
- Based on the media habits of a practice's target consumers, adjust the advertising channels to ensure the practice is reaching them in the most effective way

Measuring the true ROI on social media can be complicated. Although an exact amount may not be simple to calculate, there are many things to consider when you evaluate ROI, including:

Reach: This includes all your followers, your fans and their connections. One of your followers might have 200 followers of their own, while another has 4,000 followers. Added together, these connections can help you determine how many people you could potentially connect with on social media.

Engagement: Every time a fan "likes" your message, answers a question you've posted, or shares your message, it creates a bond with your organization and, in the long term, increases follower loyalty.

Sentiment: In addition to commenting and posting on your wall, it's essential to keep track of what fans are saying about you. Do you have a steady stream of posts about great service and short wait times? That's fantastic! Or do you have post after post about difficulty scheduling an appointment? Respond to your followers and handle the issue just as you would if a patient were at the front desk giving you feedback.

ROI needs to be measured for all other marketing efforts as well. Asking how new patients heard about the practice, or providing a written questionnaire that asks them how they discovered the practice, can help the practice determine which forms of marketing are the most effective. Then, calculate how much additional revenue was brought to the practice and subtract the cost of marketing to determine the ROI for each type of marketing effort. For example, if the practice sent 100 mailers at a cost of $200 and got two new patients, the practice needs to perform the calculations to know if the mailers were worth the effort.

Online review sites include Yelp, Healthgrades, Doctor.com, and Wellness.com. Some sites allow patients to generate reviews, while others use a combination of reviews and ratings. In other words, a review is as it sounds: sentences that indicate whether the patient was satisfied with the care they received, and if there were any perceived issues or problems. Ratings sites actually assign a rating to a physician or physician's office, usually on a scale of 1-5 or 1-10, with a low score being 1 and a high rating of 5 or 10, depending on the scale used. The ratings are usually accompanied by comments and reviews as well.

Most sites allow the practice or physician to respond to reviews. This is important when the reviews are negative. Monitoring and tracking reviews should occur on a regular basis. If most reviews are positive, an occasional negative review may not be damaging to the practice.

However, extremely negative reviews and frequent negative reviews should be taken seriously and investigated. If your practice's reviews are frequently negative when it comes to wait time, for example, it could be an indication that there is room for improvement in this area. It is also important to respond to negative reviews in the most positive way possible. That is why some practices hire outside vendors to monitor, track, and respond to online reviews. There are several companies that provide this service, and their expertise can be helpful in assuring that the practice's reputation remains positive on all fronts.

The goal of the practice website is to improve conversion rates and key performance indicators to give users the best experience, serving up the most valuable information and calls to action.

Before developing a website, reserve the practice name (and any close variation), if for no other reason than to prevent another group from using the name someday. These are called domain names, and you can reserve them for a few dollars a year.

The website is one digital access point for consumers to find information they need, and to act. A practice should:

- Understand how patients are getting to site and moving through it, and make it easier for them to find information and accomplish conversion goals
- Continually refine back- and front-end strategies to align with search engine optimization (SEO) best practices
- Understand gaps in the consumer journey
- Review and evaluate web check-ins by target market to increase completion rates

Once the practice decides to have a website, hire a professional to design and maintain the site. Security and maintenance are arguably more important than the website's design, so make sure the contract is with a firm that can handle and be accountable for those ongoing issues.

Remember that even a simple website presents the brand for the practice. While it may be prudent to start with a simple website and work up to one that is more sophisticated, the impression that the site gives potential patients is important. A professional should design the initial site with expansion in mind so the site reads and functions well.

Search Engine Optimization, or SEO, is a long-term strategy focused on improving overall visibility of a site in search engine results, which increases inbound, organic (non-paid) traffic. The practice needs to determine where it falls in a patient search. It is important for the practice to learn what search terms people are using when looking for a physician.

It is also important to note that many people who use online searches prefer to schedule an appointment online. Once the potential patient has found your practice, it is important to give that person the opportunity to schedule an appointment online. Often the person conducts the online search during the evening or on a weekend when the office may not be open. This is another reason it is critical for the practice to offer online scheduling.

As a part of the new practice launch plan, submit an application to a reputation management vendor for a new listing once the address, phone number, and go-live date are confirmed. This request will be processed, and they will schedule the listing to publish as close to the opening as possible. A practice is also at the mercy of other third-party sites (like Google, Facebook, and Yelp) to release that data, so a listing can be live through a vendor, but may take additional time to display across all review sites.

Figure 1.5

Reputation management 2.0 goals

We implement an ongoing proactive strategy to improve online reviews in both quality and quantity

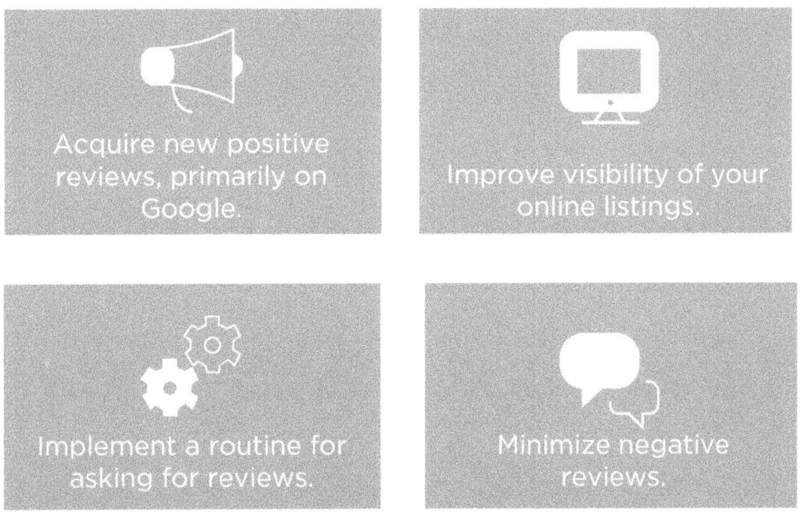

Healthcare executives who are able to promote the value of the practice, establish key relationships with clinical partners and community groups, and maintain high service and quality levels will provide the basis for personal success as well as the ongoing success of their practices.

SAMPLE QUESTIONS

1. **Which is a way practices can market to referral sources that complies with current legislation?**

   A. Meet with current providers

   B. Buy providers expensive gifts

   C. Incentivize sources with a cash bonus

   D. Refer patients to physician-owned facilities

2. **What is indicated by frequent reviews that say the medical practice's wait times are too long?**

   A. Patients don't have anything else to complain about

   B. There is room for improvement at the practice when it comes to wait time

   C. The practice is not asking for reviews at the best site

   D. Patients have become impatient

Answers: 1-A, 2-B

TASK 9: PRODUCTIVITY, COMPENSATION, AND MONITORING OF BENCHMARKS FOR PROVIDERS

Compensation of physicians and other key clinical providers is critical to the ongoing success of a medical practice. Physicians are often owners or key shareholders of the medical practice. As such, their compensation packages may vary significantly, depending on the structure of the organization and the nature of the physician's employment relationship with the organization. Therefore, determination and implementation of physician compensation is often accomplished in a significantly different manner than compensation for other practice employees. This task covers key topics in physician compensation.

The competent healthcare executive will consistently demonstrate skill in identifying types of physician compensation plans; evaluate revenue and expense allocation methods; evaluate compatibility of compensation plans with practice mission; benchmark by specialty, location, productivity, and quality; implement an effective allocation system; and comply with regulations, including Internal Revenue Service, Stark Law, and anti-kickback laws.

KEY TERM

Relative value units (RVUs): Measure of value used by Medicare for basing reimbursement to physicians.

9.1 Compensation Plans, Productivity, and Monitoring

There are many types of compensation plans for physicians. Often, compensation plans will consist of a combination of salary, incentives, and a percentage of practice profits, depending on practice ownership. Productivity has become an important measure used for determining compensation.

There are many factors that should be considered before developing a compensation plan. The compensation plan and its incentives should align with organizational objectives, individual practice objectives, larger corporate or system objectives, and input from important stakeholders.

Alignment with these objectives means that appropriate benchmarks have been gathered and key performance indicators have been chosen and are used for measuring productivity. A few of the questions the practice should be asking as it develops the plan are:

- What is your strategic plan?
- How can compensation tie directly to the strategic plan?
- What is your culture?
- What's important to you as an organization?
- How important is teamwork to the organization?

The answers to these questions determine the area the practice will want to reward with incentives. And knowing answers to these questions will help the practice develop a compensation plan that will achieve the best results in performance.

9.2 Revenue Allocation Methods

Some compensation plans, especially for independent physician-owners, assign a portion of the expenses to each physician in the practice. The proportion of expenses allotted to the physician typically corresponds to their access and productivity measures. Physicians who see more patients typically accrue more expenses. In these plans, the physicians also get a portion of the practice revenue, again, usually proportional to their productivity. Then their share of the expenses is deducted from their share of revenue.

Salary-based plans are used when the practice is owned by a corporate or larger healthcare system. Physicians may be paid an annual salary based on the market for that region, but usually the plan is a combination of an annual salary plus incentives based on measures of productivity and efficiency. Hospitalists and emergency medicine physicians may be paid an hourly rate based on their shift, with premiums paid when working the least popular shifts, such as third shift, or on weekends or holidays.

Another often-used incentive-based plan methodology looks at work relative value units, or RVUs. Each patient examination or procedure the physician performs is allotted a specified number of RVUs. The RVUs are then multiplied by a conversion factor to result in a dollar amount. The work the physician performs is considered the RVU. The more RVUs the physician completes, the higher their salary. Then the practice looks at the physician's share of expenses and the cost of malpractice insurance coverage. These are deducted from the RVUs and become the RVUs the physician will be paid for.

Physician compensation plans may also be based on panel size.[34] Attributed panels are patients that have identified the physician as their primary care doctor or patients that have been assigned to the physician or clinical team. The goal of the physician is to develop an attributed panel size that allows them to maintain a constant flow of patients while still having the ability to treat new patients and those who become more acutely ill or require more frequent services. Having the appropriate panel size ensures physicians are paid appropriately for the number of patients on their panel, and it also helps to ensure quality of care and reduces physician burnout by avoiding having too many patients.

In equal share-based plans, all physicians in the practice, department, or specific pool of physicians are paid an equal share of the revenue that has been generated after expenses have been paid. One type of physician pool would be those that are on-call, such as obstetricians.

These physicians would receive different shares for their on-call service. Physicians may also be paid shares based on their schedules or work hours.

Another factor to consider when it comes to physician compensation is how to allocate revenue and overhead when physicians' pay is based on these two financial figures. Keep in mind that practice revenue can be a combination of many different income streams, including:

- Fee-for-service collections
- Gross capitation revenue
- Net capitation revenue
- Revenue from sale of medical goods and services
- Gross revenue from other medical activities

Overhead can be a complicated figure to calculate. There are three types of overhead costs: fixed, variable, and those that should be attributed to a specific physician or cost center. Fixed expenses are those that are necessary to operate the practice with or without medical physicians or other providers, such as rent and utility costs. Variable costs such as medical supplies will change according to how many patients are seen. Wages and payroll taxes are examples of the third kind of overhead, as they are specific to a physician or cost center. The question becomes: What is a fair way to allocate revenue and overhead? Two primary ways to consider overhead, for example, include:

1. Allocate overhead equally among physicians, because all have equal access to facilities
2. Allocate overhead based on production

There are several methods practices can use to determine revenue allocation. Revenue can be based on collections, gross or net charges, RVUs, or a hybrid of all of these measures:

- Work relative value units
- Collections or charges (gross or net); collections include all funds received on billed charges; since not all billed charges are paid immediately, practices may base compensation on actual money collected
- Equal share (or equal based on physicians taking calls)
- Team-based (teams of physicians and mid-level providers)
- Allocation of ancillary revenue pool (Stark compliant)
- Participation in alternative payment systems
- Hybrid of all of the above

9.3 Expense Allocation Methods

The primary ways to allocate expenses to physicians as part of their compensation plan include:

- Per capita (each physician pays an equal share)
- Patient encounter volume (the physician's share depends on the number of patient encounters)
- Work relative value units (the physician's share depends on the RVUs produced)

- Percent of charges or collections (the physician's share is tied to the percent of charges or collections brought into the practice)
- Square footage (the physician's share coordinates with the square footage used)
- Physician benefits pooled or individually assigned
- Hybrid of the above methods

Physicians' compensation plans may also include a number of nonproduction incentives that should coordinate with the strategic plan and mission as well as other services the physician or practice provides. These can include:

- Quality incentives
- Corporate citizenship incentives
- Patient satisfaction incentives
- Teaching and research incentives

Figure 1.6

Plan	Pros	Cons
Straight salary	Easiest to understand and use	Does not encourage quality improvements or cost savings
Salary plus bonus	May encourage quality and productivity improvements	Bonus criteria must be carefully chosen
Equal shares	Physicians typically watch resource use	Can create conflict
Pay for performance	Incentivizes performance and quality objectives	Complex and more difficult to track and administer
Productivity-based	Extra efforts and cost savings are rewarded	May create competitive environment among physicians

9.4 Providers' Employment Contracts

If the practice needs physician compensation contracts, preparing and executing them correctly are essential.

Working with legal counsel, the group should develop a standard physician compensation contract. You can customize the contract, especially the compensation section, for each new physician. This method allows you to create uniform contracts without them being identical. Counsel should also prepare a standard contract for part-time employees, and for advanced practice providers. Your counsel for this project must be an attorney with extensive experience in healthcare transaction law and healthcare contract law. Only a specialist will do.

Once the contract forms are developed, avoid the temptation to skip the involvement of your legal counsel in future physician contracts. At a minimum, your counsel should review each negotiated contract before it is signed. Compared to the original contract drafting, this review should be less expensive. Whether the practice attorney is involved in negotiations may depend on the preferences of the parties.

Contracts are written to cover these situations and information:[35]

Full Partner, Senior Physician: These are physicians who may have founded or started the practice or who have worked there for many years and earned a partnership. These contracts will consist of more benefits and privileges than the other contract types.

Associate or New Physician: These are contracts for new physicians joining the practice. The practice may offer part ownerships or partnerships to new physicians, or they may be considered employees.

Locum tenens or fill-in physicians: Contracts for physicians that may work at the practice during times when the regular practice physicians are taking time off for various reasons. They may see patients for a few days, weeks, or for months at a time.

Special Circumstance: There may be times when the practice requires extra coverage on a part-time or on-call basis. Contracts will need to provide details of the circumstances, maximum and minimum number of hours required, etc.

Employment status should be spelled out in the contract, explaining whether the physician is considered an owner, partner, employee, or independent contractor.

9.5 Credentialing

Providers must go through the credentialing process in the hospital setting as a separate entity. Hospital credentialing involves verification and review of the applicant's education, training and experience, and licensing to practice medicine. This is performed by the hospital committee that also oversees assignment of provider privileges. Credentialing is the first step for a hospital to grant a provider privileges authorizing them to provide services at the hospital.

9.6 Patient Relations

Patient relations are a critical part of a successful medical practice. Ensuring that patients are satisfied with the care and treatment they receive while visiting the facility and that any complaints or concerns are addressed should be part of every physician's job. Physicians should actively participate in service recovery plans in cases where patients are dissatisfied with care or had unusually long wait times or other unsatisfactory experiences. Compensation plans should include the expectation that physicians will participate in and act on service recovery plans. Some compensation plans also include metrics of the patient experience, which means they might receive bonuses or incentives based on patients' reports of their experiences with the both the physician and the practice. Patient experience is usually measured by inviting patients to complete a survey following visits.

9.7 Provider Benchmarking

Benchmarks consist of key performance indicators associated with each item being measured. Production benchmarks could include any or all of the following:

- RVUs
- Visits (number of visits per day, per week, per month, etc.)
- Hours (hours worked throughout the week, month, year, etc.)

Benchmarks are ideal measures the practice would like to achieve, and they are gathered using national data such as data the MGMA provides. Benchmarks then should be set as a threshold and used to determine at which measures the physician receives an incentive, bonus, or other form of compensation.

Compensation itself can take many forms, from a biweekly salary, a monthly salary, annual cash incentive payments, medical director compensation, additional on-call pay, and incentives for patient survey participation and results.

The effective management of physician compensation is complex, requiring sophisticated interpersonal and technical skills. The practice executive demonstrates leadership in this area by identifying and implementing compensation packages that support the mission of the practice as well as the motivation of physicians and the quality of patient care delivery.

SAMPLE QUESTIONS

1. **Which sentence describes an equal share-based physician compensation plan?**

   A. Physicians are paid according to attributed panel size

   B. Physicians are paid an annual salary based on the regional market

   C. All physicians in the practice are paid an equal share of the revenue after expenses have been paid

   D. Physicians are paid shares of the revenue based on their schedules or work hours

2. **Which is a way expenses can be allocated when calculating physician compensation?**

   A. Square footage

   B. Panel size

   C. Participation in alternate payment systems

   D. Participation in service recovery programs

Answers: 1-C, 2-A

TASK 10: QUALITY INITIATIVES

Quality management programs are used to reduce errors and improve patient care. Knowing that patient experience influences outcomes provides an inherent motivation to reassess processes that enhance care delivery. These efforts increase provider satisfaction and improve practice culture. Efforts to improve patient care and reduce errors start with a quality management process and roll outward.

Quality management initiatives help professionals design, implement, and maintain measurement activities, and administrative policies and procedures that ensure patient safety and the consistent delivery of quality care. In practical terms, that means:[36]

- Using analytical processes, such as Lean or total quality improvement programs, to improve interaction and communication between all team members
- Creating internal tracking so that medical practice groups can compare their practices with others on quality, safety, and cost benchmarks
- Establishing, evaluating, and enforcing standards for quality

Quality initiatives should be a part of a medical practice's daily operations. No matter how smoothly a practice may be running, there is always room for improvements in quality. Medical practices should identify and plan for quality initiatives on at least a yearly basis.

In addition, the U.S. Department of Health and Human Services, along with the Institute of Medicine recommend that healthcare facilities, including medical practices, engage in quality initiatives to improve their service delivery approach or systems of care. They recommend all quality initiatives follow four key principles:[37]

- Function as systems and processes
- Focus on patients
- Focus on being part of the team
- Focus on use of the data

10.1 Utilization Management

According to the Utilization Review Accreditation Commission (URAC),[38] utilization management is defined as evaluating the medical necessity, appropriateness, and efficiency of healthcare services, procedures, and facilities. For medical practices, this means examining the medical necessity, appropriateness, and efficiency of the services and procedures they perform. Quality initiatives that focus on utilization management may examine one or all of these factors.

The Centers for Medicare and Medicaid Services (CMS) defines medical necessity as "services or supplies that are proper and needed for the diagnosis or treatment of a medical condition, are provided for the diagnosis, direct care, and treatment of a medical condition, meet the standards of good medical practice in the local area, and aren't mainly for the convenience of the patient or doctor."[39]

Quality initiatives that focus on medical necessity and appropriateness should consider three perspectives:

- **Prospective Reviews:** Review of medical necessity prior to the procedure, treatment, or service being provided
- **Concurrent Reviews:** Review of medical necessity decisions while procedure, service, or treatment is being provided
- **Retrospective Reviews:** Review of medical necessity decisions after procedure, service, or treatment has been provided

Medical necessity means the procedure, treatment, or service is appropriate, justifiable, and reimbursable. It is important that all initiatives are based on a clinically sound foundation and never on costs alone. These reviews can include:

- Level of care determinations
- Assessment of any delays in care
- Assessment for medical necessity and appropriateness throughout progression of care
- Accurate documentation
- Review of documentation
- Second-level physician reviews
- Clinical documentation improvements

Prior authorization occurs when the practice schedules a treatment or procedure for a patient and submits the information to the payer for approval prior to performing the procedure. When the payer grants approval, the procedure or treatment is considered medically necessary and reimbursable. One way for practices to determine if the services and treatments they are offering patients are considered medically necessary is to find industry benchmarks for prior authorization and compare the practice's rate of prior authorization to the benchmarks. Then the practice can determine if its prior authorization rate needs to be improved.

Benchmarking and analysis are essential components of quality initiatives. Benchmarking and quality initiatives have been launched to control healthcare costs, structure the management of risk and quality of care, and to satisfy patients' expectations. Benchmarking has taken many different forms over the last few decades. In general, though, benchmarks either provide a starting point for improvement programs, or a goal for practices to achieve. Benchmarks may either be determined at the practice, or by using available industry measures. For example, one measure of quality is patient wait time. An industry benchmark of best practice wait time for patients could be the goal the practice wants to achieve. Then, the practice gathers its own data to determine their average wait time. This information provides a baseline. Then, the practice can adjust the benchmark if needed. Clinical practice benchmarking involves structured comparisons of best practices in clinical care and processes based on quality assessment, and is integrated within a continuous quality improvement (CQI) approach.

According to the Agency for Healthcare Research and Quality (AHRQ), practices should identify appropriate benchmarks in comparison to the items they wish to improve. Practices can generate benchmarks from similar practices in the same physical area or by comparing their benchmarks to a larger group of practices across the country. Benchmarks may also be drawn from standards set by an authoritative body such as CMS.

Practices may also find good sources of benchmarks when data are required for reporting to federal agencies and funders such as the Health Resources and Services Administration's Uniform Data System reports required from Federally Qualified Health Centers (FQHC). National professional associations and the National Committee on Quality Assurance (NCQA) are other potential resources for benchmarking. Practices may also find state and local health agencies and public health agencies good sources of benchmarks.

10.2 Patient Education

Patient education is vital to the quality of healthcare. Educating patients about their health status, current medical conditions, and how to improve their quality of health is vital for compliance with physician recommendations. Studies have shown that the average patient retains just 50% of what the physician communicates to them. Using quality initiatives to better educate patients can lead to better clinical outcomes and quality of care.

Patient education improvements should look at three parts of healthcare delivery:

- Communication of diagnosis
- Management of condition and treatment protocols
- Follow-up at the end of the patient visit

Quality initiatives related to patient education could include the following:

Staff training and education: Train staff to ensure they are able to communicate clearly and precisely, when appropriate, about the patient's diagnosis. Train staff to recognize when a patient may not understand what is being communicated.

Technology: Offering technologies to improve patient understanding could include specific apps for patients to monitor vital healthcare statuses, reference accurate and reliable videos that provide information about the patient's condition, and provide personalized information electronically.

High-quality educational resources: Practices can find high-quality educational resources through many different sources, such as universities, research centers, and associations such as the American Heart Association and the American Lung Association. Taking the time to provide these resources to patients and their families can lead to better outcomes.

Workflows: Workflows should be redesigned to include patient education. This could mean ensuring that resources are provided, as well as allowing additional time with a provider for the patient to ask questions.

- Critical care
- Other services, such as home services, case management, and telemedicine

The code may be an E&M code, a procedure code, or both. When these areas are fully documented, they reflect the physicians' work and help determine reimbursement amounts. The practice needs to ensure that the codes accurately describe the services provided and the related diagnosis.

In order to receive full and appropriate reimbursement for services, the practice should implement policies and procedures to ensure that it accurately bills all services performed. The process of capturing (recording) the charge for the service rendered to the patient and then billing and collecting for it might seem straightforward, but it is error prone in many practices and requires clear processes and discipline.

Patient Encounter Records

Failure to document a service means not being able to bill for that service. The encounter form is an internal document used to generate the bill and can be customized for the practice to include the current procedure and diagnosis codes used most frequently by the physicians.[1] The form becomes a document of the encounter that can be used to initiate the billing process, culminating in the super bill, an itemized form that details services provided to a patient. It is the main data source for creation of a healthcare claim, which will be submitted to payers.

Physicians practice in many locations, including hospitals. Patient demographics and hospital charges can be captured via an interface between the hospital data system and the practice data system.

Electronic Claims Processing

Electronic claims processing is the electronic submission of claims to payers or clearinghouses that reformat the data and retransmit it to the appropriate insurance company or fiscal intermediary. Benefits include:

- Edit (and correct) claims before submitting them to payers
- Easily generate productivity reports
- Reduce rebilling
- Improve cost-effectiveness in billing

Payment Posting

Third-party payers provide an explanation of benefits (EOB) or electronic remittance advice (ERA) when they pay claims. The EOB explains how the payer computed the amount it paid (or did not pay) for the claim. This information is generally itemized by CPT code or description and includes the:

- Gross amount of claim
- Amount allowable

Literacy: Practices should also check for patient health literacy, which means to discover how well informed patients are about their health and any condition they have. Assumptions should never be made about how much a patient does or does not know. Physicians should make the effort to improve the health literacy of the practice's patients. This can include providing ongoing tips and suggestions for better health.

Standards: Practices may also use CMS and Joint Commission standards to improve patient education.

10.3 Quality Incentives

Other reasons practices launch quality programs is to ensure they meet quality standards and incentives derived from national and federal organizations such as CMS and the Joint Commission. While not all practices are required to participate in these programs, most do, and those that do will need to show they meet quality standards to receive any incentives.

The National Committee for Quality Assurance (NCQA) is a national association with a mission to improve the quality of healthcare. It achieves this mission through several different programs for practices, hospitals, and other providers. NCQA currently offers seven programs for physician practices, which also lead to certification by NCQA. Most of these programs seek to make all care patient-centered.

The Healthcare Effectiveness Data and Information Set (HEDIS) is another program designed and administered by NCQA. NCQA collects data from health plans and other healthcare organizations using more than 90 measures and across six domains:[40]

- Effectiveness of care
- Access/availability of care
- Experience of care
- Utilization and risk-adjusted utilization
- Health plan descriptive information
- Measures collected using electronic clinical data systems

NCQA performs regular audits of this information to ensure its accuracy, and it publishes them in different forms for the healthcare industry to use.

10.4 Coordination of Care

Coordination of care is an additional aspect of care that is often ripe for quality improvements. Often when ancillary services, specialist encounters, or similar services are required of patients, the practice may not have the systems in place to guarantee that the patient receives those services. Practices should examine the systems they currently have in place when recommending:

- Ancillary services
- Specialist visits
- Home health services

- Therapy of any kind
- Education
- Hospitalization

First, the practice should do a thorough examination of the referral and authorization process. How are patients referred to other providers? What information are they given? How is the practice notified that the patient has acted on the referral? What patient follow-ups are in place?

When the treatment or procedure is complete, the practice should be informed of the transfer of the patient to another facility, if needed, as well as the patient's discharge. The practice should be aware of any additional follow-up appointments that are required post-discharge and encourage patients to complete them.

Patient flow should be intensively managed by the practice for quality reasons. Patient visits per day, week, month, and year should be tracked per practice, per physician or provider, or per team. Practices should examine the length of consultation and exam, how often exam rooms are underutilized, and other similar measures. Patient flow issues can indicate several different quality issues that may need to be improved.

Additional quality improvement areas practices should consider include the following:

Government or insurance mandated processes and forms, such as HIPAA notices: What process is in place to meet the requirements? Has the practice gathered data to ensure it is meeting them? What quality improvements could be made to ensure they are met 100% of the time?

Interoperability: Are health information systems working together to inform healthcare decisions? Are systems providing all the information that is needed across teams and providers?

Records management: Are healthcare records accurate, complete, and do they meet privacy requirements? Are medical records updated in a timely manner?

Translation services: Are patients whose first language is not English provided with a translator or interpreter? What system does the practice have in place to ensure an interpreter is provided when needed? Are important patient documents available in languages that are prevalent in the practice's community?

To ensure quality of care and best possible patient outcomes, these questions and others should be answered, and quality initiatives put in place as needed.

Quality initiatives have been instituted in the healthcare field since the 1980s and 1990s. Initiatives have become more complex, but are considered essential for many reasons, including providing quality care and improving patient outcomes. Nearly every aspect of practice operations could be the target of quality improvement. It is important for practices to first obtain quality benchmarks, gather data, and compare practice measures against benchmarks to prioritize quality initiatives. Quality improvement programs also result in a more positive work environment and higher levels of employee retention.

SAMPLE QUESTIONS

1. **Why do practices implement quality improvement programs?**
   A. To attract more patients
   B. To reduce errors and improve patient care
   C. To reduce costs
   D. To improve revenue flow

2. **Why is patient education important?**
   A. It leads to an improved reputation in the community
   B. It is mandated by law
   C. It leads to an increase in the number of patient visits
   D. It is vital for compliance with physician recommendations

Answers: 1-B, 2-D

OPERATIONS MANAGEMENT QUIZ

1. Which is a definition of an organization's mission?

A. The mission is the organization's precise statement of purpose

B. The mission describes the organization's values

C. The mission describes the organization's vision

D. The mission is the organization's goals for the next five years

2. What happens during the planning phase in project management?

A. You conduct market research

B. You determine costs

C. You find background information

D. You create a step-by-step plan for executing the project

3. Which is a factor to consider when choosing a location for a medical practice?

A. Where it is in relation to most staff members' homes

B. Where it is in relation to the city's downtown region

C. Where it is in relation to feeder streets and highways

D. Where it is in relation to other medical practices

4. Which is one of the 4 A's of marketing for medical practices?

A. Accuracy

B. Advertising

C. Advice

D. Access

ANSWERS

1-A. The mission is the organization's precise statement of purpose.

2-D. Planning should be transparent, meaning all team members, stakeholders, and the project sponsor should clearly see that the plan is designed to meet the goals and that there are no hidden objectives.

3-C. Factors include being in the approximate center of your market area, being close to your primary hospital, being in a high-traffic, high-visibility area, and in a location with easy access to major feeder streets and highways.

4-D. The four A's of marketing for medical practices are access, availability, accountability, and accommodation.

Notes

1. "Policy and Procedure Considerations for Health Information Exchange Organizations, The American Health Information Management Association, http://bok.ahima.org/doc?oid=107715#.XwslpZNKifV.
2. John M. Bryson, *Strategic Planning for Public and Nonprofit Organizations: A Guide to Strengthening and Sustaining Organizational Achievement* (San Francisco: Jossey-Bass, 2004).
3. Russell L. Ackoff, *A Concept of Corporate Planning* (New York: Wiley Interscience, 1970); Henry Mintzberg, *The Rise and Fall of Strategic Planning* (New York: Simon and Schuster, 1994), 11.
4. Bryson, *Strategic Planning.*
5. Carter McNamara, *Field Guide to Nonprofit Strategic Planning and Facilitation* (Minneapolis, MN: Authenticity Consulting LLC, 2000).
6. Linda E. Swayne, Peter M. Ginter, and W. Jack Duncan, *The Physician Strategist: Setting a Strategic Direction for Your Practice* (Chicago: Irwin Professional Publishing, 1996).
7. "Start Your Project Right: A Complete Guide to Project Initiation," The Digital Project Manager, http://thedigitalprojectmanager.com.
8. "Gantt Chart Template for Excel," Vertex42, http://vertex42.com/ExcepTemplates/excel-gantt-chart.html.
9. "Project Management in Healthcare," Clearpointstrategy.com, http://clearpointstrategy.com/project-management-in-healthcare.
10. Ibid.
11. Ibid.
12. Ibid.
13. O'Brien, Daniel, Jon Leibowitz, Russell Anello, *How Group Purchasing Organizations Reduce Healthcare Procurement Costs in a Highly Competitive Market,* June 2017.
14. "3 Different Types of Commercial Real Estate Leases," 42Floors, https://42floors.com/edu/basics/types-of-commercial-real-estate-leases.
15. "Legal Forms of Organization for a Medical Practice," *Medical Practice and the Law,* Medscape, http://medscape.com/courses/section/870049.
16. "Limited Liability Company," Entrepreneur Encyclopedia, *Entrepreneur,* http://entrepreneur.com/encyclopedia/limited-liability-company.
17. "Legal Forms of Organization for a Medical Practice," *Medical Practice and the Law.*

18. Torrey, Trisha. "How Health Insurance Co-ops Work," Verywellhealth.com, http://verywellhealth.com/what-is-a-health-insurance-co-op-2615262, updated February 26, 2020.
19. Nick Hernandez, "What Medical Practices Should Know about Joint Ventures," *The Doctor Weighs In*, June 8, 2018.
20. Jenny Gold, "Accountable Care Organizations Explained," *Kaiser Health News*, Kaiser Family Foundation.
21. Peter R. Kongstvedt, David W. Plocher, and Jean C. Stanford, "Integrated Health Care Delivery Systems," in *Essentials of Managed Health Care*, 4th ed., ed. Peter R. Kongstvedt (Gaithersburg, MD: Aspen, 2001), 31-62.
22. Alan M. Zuckerman, "Strategic Alliances and Joint Ventures: Why Make When You Can Buy?" *Healthcare Financial Management* 59, no. 8 (2005): 122-124.
23. Kongstvedt et al., "Integrated Health Care Delivery Systems."
24. Sarah Stubee, "Key Considerations for every physician before acquiring a practice," PhysiciansPractice.com, http://physicianspractice.com/view/key-considerations-every-physician-acquiring-practice.
25. S. Cohen, "Emerging Benefits of Integrated IT Systems," *Healthcare Executive* 20, no. 5 (2005): 14-18.
26. C. Pope, "The Hereafter: Why IT Security Matters to Your Practice Even After the HIPAA Security Rule Deadline," *MGMA Connection* 5, no. 6 (2005): 36-41.
27. Ibid.
28. Department of Health and Human Services, 45 C.F.R. pt. 162, HIPAA Administrative Simplification: Standard Unique Health Identifier for Health Care Providers; Final Rule, *Fed. Reg.* (May 31, 2002), 3433-3469.
29. A.T. Eliscu, "Marketing for Straight A's? How One Practice Created a Customer-Service Brand Identity," *MGMA Connexion* 8, no. 5 (May-June 2008): 50-53, 1.
30. "Definition of Marketing: Marketing Research," American Marketing Association, 1995, www.marketingpower.com.
31. Meir Liraz, *Small Business Management: Essential Ingredients for Success*, Best Business Books, 1998, www.bizmove.com/free-pdf-download/small-busi nessmanagement.pdf.
32. E. Jerome McCarthy, *Basic Marketing: A Managerial Approach* (Homewood, IL: R.D. Irwin, 1960).
33. "GTP Organizer Training: Training Guide #7: Organizational Structure and Culture," Gather the People, 2004, www.gatherthepeople.org/ Downloads/007_STRUCTURE_CULTURE.pdf.
34. "Identifying the Optimal Panel Sizes for Primary Care Physicians," Steps Forward: Workflow and Process, American Medical Association, http://edhub.ama-assn.org/steps-forward/module/2702760.
35. Bruce A. Johnson and Deborah Walker Keegan, *Physician Compensation Plans: State-of-the-Art Strategies* (Englewood, CO: MGMA, 2009).
36. W. Edwards Deming, *Out of the Crisis* (Cambridge, MA: Massachusetts Institute of Technology, Center for Advanced Engineering Studies, 1990), 166.
37. Agency for Healthcare Research and Quality, http://ahrq.gov.
38. India Watson, "The Utilization Review Process and the Origins of Medical Necessity," MCG Health, Heast Health Network, June 21, 2018, http://mcg.com/blog/2018/06/21/utilization-review-medical-necessity.
39. "Medical Necessity," The Center for Medicare and Medicaid Services, http://cms.gov.
40. "HEDIS and Performance Measurement," National Committee for Quality Assurance, http://ncqa.org/hedis.

Chapter 2

Financial Management

How do you develop and maintain financial systems to ensure a profitable practice? Financial management is both a very broad and very deep process. Financial management in a medical group requires skills in accounting, budgeting, revenue cycle management, and financial analysis. Questions on the American College of Medical Practice Executives objective exam focus on the issues that healthcare executives commonly face while implementing these important functions.

The key knowledge and tasks in this area are:

1. Revenue Cycle
2. Cash Flow Management
3. Accounts Payable Management
4. Payroll Management
5. Budget Creation and Management
6. Financial Reporting
7. Audit Management
8. Corporate Tax Reporting

TASK 1: REVENUE CYCLE

The billing and collection process is complex, with multiple payers, varying fee schedules, numerous rules and regulations, compliance challenges, and many opportunities for practices to fail to receive payment for services.

The key skills and knowledge necessary to successfully manage the financial health of a medical practice include:

- Managing front-end operations, including scheduling, insurance verification, authorizations, copayments, and collection of deductibles
- Overseeing medical record documentation, charge capture, and coding
- Managing charge audit
- Submitting claims and resolving edits
- Implementing accounts receivable follow-up and refund processes
- Monitoring and reporting key metrics
- Analyzing reimbursements and reviewing contracts
- Managing and negotiating payer contracts
- Managing charge masters and payment schedules
- Managing payer credentialing

KEY TERMS

Accounts receivable (A/R): The open amounts (debts) owed to the organization by other entities.

Coordination of benefits: The process whereby two or more insurance companies or insuring entities apportion each one's share of the responsibility for payment of a claim for healthcare services provided to a client who is insured by them.

Contractual allowance or contractual adjustment: Write-offs resulting from payers paying less than billed charges.

Current Procedural Terminology (CPT): Coding developed and maintained by the American Medical Association. A five-digit numeric code assigned to different physician actions.

Electronic Remittance Advice (ERA): An electronic data interchange (EDI) version of a medical insurance payment explanation. It provides details about providers' claims payment, and if the claims are denied, it would then contain the required explanations. The explanations include the denial codes and the descriptions, which present at the bottom of ERA.

Explanation of Benefits (EOB): A document provided to the patient by the insurance company following a healthcare service for which a claim was submitted. The EOB gives information about how an insurance claim was paid on the patient's behalf — if applicable — and how much the patient is responsible for.

Healthcare Common Procedure Coding System (HCSPCS): Used by the Centers for Medicare & Medicaid Services (CMS) to bill Medicare, Medicaid and many other third-party payers.

(continued on next page)

ICD-10: International Classification of Diseases, Tenth Revision

Resource-Based Relative Value System (RBRVS): The physician payment system used by the Centers for Medicare & Medicaid Services (CMS) and most other payers.

Reasonable and customary fee: The fee charged for a specified procedure by a particular type of healthcare provider practicing within a specified geographic area. Insurance companies often use "reasonable and customary fee" to define the amount they will cover for a specific procedure.

Revenue cycle management: All administrative and clinical functions that contribute to the capture, management, and collection of patient service revenue.

Relative value unit (RVU): Payer-assigned value to a particular service and tied to a CPT code.

1.1 Lifecycle of a Claim

Registration

As a first step, the patient information should be entered in the system to include patient demographic and identifying information, such as name and address, as well as the reason for the visit. The practice should capture insurance and patient payment information at this time, too.

Coding

Every code that is billed should be adequately documented by the physician in the medical record using ICD-10-CM CPT codes (or ASA units for anesthesia), along with at least one corresponding diagnosis code.

Medicare uses the RBRVS, which assigns relative values to most of the CPT codes based on the resources that a physician typically uses to perform the service. This forms the basis for payment. In addition, HCPCS codes are used to identify services not fully described in the CPT system, such as ambulance transportation, injections, durable medical equipment, and supplies or services that have not yet been assigned CPT codes.

Evaluation and management (E&M) codes are listed in the AMA CPT codebooks and represent the cognitive services that physicians perform. Each of these areas has as many as five levels of care, from simple to complex. The CPT E&M codes apply to:

- Office visits
- Hospital visits
- Consultations
- Emergency services

- Amount excluded and reason it was excluded
- Amount of patient responsibility and explanation (i.e., copayment, deductible, or coinsurance)
- Amount paid or denial of the claim with the reason for the denial

When received, the payment should be posted to ensure that contractual allowances and allowable amounts on the EOB are correct, according to the practice's contract. Most practice management systems allow the practice to enter its fee schedules by payer into the system. The practice needs to ensure that the fee schedules in its system are current or this tool will not be effective. The system should signal any incorrect amounts, and a staff member should follow up on errors.

When a denial occurs, it is vital that it be posted with the reason for denial to assure effective follow-up (see upcoming Denial Management section).

If there is a remaining patient due balance after posting the payment, a bill is sent to the patient.

Insurance Follow-Up

When practices submit claims electronically, transmission and acceptance reports create an audit trail indicating which claims were successfully transmitted and received by the payer and which were not. Practices need to ensure that a billing staff person is responsible for monitoring these reports and correcting claims that did not process or transmit correctly.

If the contractual allowance or payment is incorrect, a staff member should be responsible for following up on errors. Failure to write off a contractual allowance for a payer with whom the practice participates is a violation of the practice's contract with that payer.

The practice should audit or review the work on a regular basis to ensure that the contractual allowances are being handled properly. For example, if staff members write off patient responsibility or adjustments made by payers with whom the practice does not participate, the practice loses that money.

Auditing Payments

Managing the individual claim EOBs is one way to improve collections. An internal audit program that supplements EOB processing is another method for improvement.

There are four steps to consider when structuring the auditing process for the practice. They are:

1. Organize your contract files. Files should be readily accessible with easy access for auditors.
2. Identify and monitor key indicators from the contract; both financial and operational.
3. Track and document discrepancies.
4. Prepare to mediate, arbitrate, or litigate.

Denial Management

Denial management addresses the nonpayment of claims (the practice bill) by insurance companies and is one of the more complex parts of A/R collections.

- The first step is to review the EOBs and categorize the reasons for denials given by insurance companies. Payers can then be benchmarked against each other to determine trends and patterns.
- The practice's denial codes should be broad enough to segregate denials caused by practice coding issues and those that are payer driven.
- Inappropriate payer denials should be managed aggressively.
- Finally, be aware of contractual and state requirements and make sure you collect what is due.

The practice should have a process and staff assigned to pursue denied claims and to make sure there are no internal systemic problems in the practice's billing process.

Withholds, which apply to capitation payments, occur when the payer retains part of the payment for a period of time, to be returned at a later date if certain payer and provider objectives are met. If withholds cannot be avoided, the practice should track how much has been withheld over the agreed-upon time span, and follow up with requests for payment.

Collections

Financial responsibility: Commercial and government payers often do not pay the entire allowable fee. The patient must frequently bear a portion of the cost in the form of a copayment, coinsurance, or deductible.

Secondary insurance coverage: Some patients are covered by more than one payer. When a patient has two insurance policies, one is the primary insurance and the other is secondary. In fact, in some cases patients can even have a third, or tertiary insurance. In a process called coordination of benefits, the practice should bill the primary insurance first. After the primary insurance has paid or settled, the practice should then bill the secondary insurance.

The practice needs to ensure that its staff (or billing company) resolves overpayments that result in credit balances and refund the proper payer within a reasonable period of time (this may be defined in the practice's contract with the payer). Failure to do so may lead to compliance problems and breach of contract with the payer.

A large number of unresolved credit balances can create misleading A/R indicators. This is because practices often compute their A/R net of credit balances. If those credit balances are large and old, they decrease not only the total balance of the A/R (and the related days in A/R) but the aging percentage of the old balances. Thus, the metrics mislead the practice as to the true potential for improved financial performance from revenue cycle initiatives.

It is important that the practice have a payment policy and that staff is familiar with the policy. Ideally, payment is collected at the time of service. At a minimum, the policy should:

- Require that patients make their copayments at the time of service
- Clearly state what the practice will do if the patient does not pay
    - Will the patient be rescheduled?
    - Is partial payment accepted?
- Require payment of past due balances within 30 days
    - Spell out consequences if patients fail to pay past balances
    - Provide examples of an acceptable partial payment
    - Provide the circumstances (if any) under which the practice will agree to an extended payment plan with the patient
- Identify non-covered services and how payments are handled for those services.

Collections may be handled internally or outsourced. Regardless, individuals reaching out to patients must be sensitive to the patient and have a clear understanding of what types of payment plans are acceptable to the practice. Anyone working in collections needs to understand what is and is not acceptable regarding write-offs to be consistent with anti-kickback and Stark laws.

Should the practice decide to outsource collections, factors to consider when selecting a collection agency are:

1) Their approach to patients, as they represent the practice and may dissuade patients from seeking care with the practice if they have a negative experience with the collection agency
2) Their collection performance
3) The commission charged

1.2 Payer Reimbursement Policies

Getting paid presents special challenges for physician practices, whether it is collecting from the patient or a third-party payer. Contractual allowables are based on each payer's contract and, in some cases, the provider manual or other documents referenced in the contract. The healthcare executive and the billing staff need to be familiar with the various methods that third-party payers use to pay providers.

The practice must submit bills (or claims) to the payers in a standardized format, in compliance with government regulations and payer policies. Practices should keep current with all guidelines.

Payers, including the Medicare program, apply various payment guidelines to reimburse physicians for services they render to patients. These guidelines rely on published numerical codes that a provider enters on an electronic encounter form to indicate the medical diagnosis and the resulting services, procedures, or supplies that are rendered. Practices must establish standards for proper documentation and coding to ensure that billing is accurate and complete. Improper coding and documentation can cause overpayments, underpayments, and denials of claims.

Private insurance companies may set payment policies within the broader outlines of state and federal regulations. The healthcare executive must ensure that the practice follows the reimbursement, coding, and collection policies of its many private insurance payers.

Discounted Fee-for-Service

Beginning with the advent of managed care in the 1980s, the most common method commercial payers used to control costs was to negotiate with providers, who agreed to charge less than their usual fee in exchange for participation with that payer.

The Medicare fee schedule is based on a comprehensive study of the relative cost of the resources used (including malpractice, practice expense, and work of the provider) to provide each medical service a value as compared to other services. This was called the *resource-based relative value system* (RBRVS).

The RBRVS assigns relative values to most of the CPT codes. The values are based on the resources that a physician typically uses to perform the service.

The RBRVS uses relative values — nonmonetary, relative units of measure — for most of the CPT (CPT-4) codes. It converts these relative values into dollar amounts by applying a conversion factor.

To develop its own relative value units (RVUs), a practice can extract procedure code data from its billing system and relate those data to the relative value weights for each procedure as assigned by the Medicare RBRVS. RVUs are determined by three components:

1. Physician's work: The amount of time, skill, training, and intensity necessary to perform a given procedure. The work RVU accounts for 53% of the total RVU.
2. Practice expense: Intended to recognize costs such as rent, equipment and supplies, consulting and professional services, and staff salaries.
3. Malpractice expense: Refers to the liability expenditures borne by or on behalf of the provider (just 3% of the total).

Each component is multiplied by a factor known as the Geographic Practice Cost Index, or GPCI, to account for variations in living and business costs across the country.

Percentage of Medicare

Many commercial carriers base contract payments on the Medicare fee schedule to simplify reimbursement. Practices can negotiate a percentage of the expected Medicare payment (typically greater than 100% of Medicare) for the same services according to the RBRVS schedule.

Capitation

Some managed care organizations use *capitation* or prepaid services, to reimburse for services. Under this model, the payer and the provider negotiate a fixed periodic payment (usually monthly) paid to the provider to provide specific healthcare services to an attributed patient population.

Under capitation, the practice is paid whether it sees the patients or not; consequently, lower volumes of services are more profitable; higher volume results in higher variable costs. Under advanced forms of capitation, providers assume financial risk for the patient population. This is sometimes referred to as *global capitation*. The provider group's reimbursement includes payment for the total delivery of healthcare services within a specified scope.

Value-Based Care

Value-based care, also known as pay for performance, or P4P, ties physician payments and other healthcare provider payments to defined performance standards.

Providers can participate in Medicare's MACRA either as a member of an Advanced Alternative Payment Model (APM) or using the Merit-based Incentive Payment System (MIPS). Advanced APMs operate as either a medical home model under CMS innovation center authority or require members to assume significant financial risk.

Providers participating in an Advanced APM may potentially receive a 5% bonus and are exempt from MIPS.

Eligible providers (those who are eligible clinician types and meet certain minimum volume thresholds) who do not participate in an Advanced APM are included in MIPS. For MIPS, providers report under four categories:

1. **Quality** *(This replaced the former PQRS discussed above)*
2. **Promoting interoperability** *(This replaced the Medicare EHR Incentive Program, also known as Meaningful Use)*
3. **Improvement Activities** *(For this new category, participants self-report from an inventory of activities that improve the care process, patient engagement and/or access to care)*
4. **Cost** *(This is calculated by CMS based upon claims)*

Private payers may also have quality reporting programs. These take several common forms. For example, a typical program will reward a physician with a bonus depending on how well they perform on certain quality measures and/or may use the Healthcare Effectiveness Data and Information Set (HEDIS) standards to rate the physician or provider, according to the National Committee for Quality Assurance (NCQA).

- Quality outcomes and screening
- Patient engagement (e.g., satisfaction scores)
- Efficiency (e.g., hospitalization rates)

These metrics can make up 20% or more of the total reimbursement. If a practice elects to participate in a quality care program, it will need to ensure that it provides all the necessary information to the payer.

1.3 Payer Types

Medical practices collect money from a variety of payers. These include commercial payers, the government, workers' compensation, and the patients themselves.

Keep in mind, due to the large volume of business with Medicare and other governmental payers that require discounted fee schedules and discounted fee-for-service contracts with commercial payers, today's medical practices find that they do a considerable amount of business at lower rates than their billed charges. The write-offs are called *contractual allowances or contractual adjustments.*

Managed Care

Physicians historically had considerable autonomy over treatment options and the amount they charged for their services. Now, the commercial payers utilize policies to manage the way physicians and other providers practice medicine. The methods that those organizations use to manage care include:

- Requiring that certain surgeries be performed on an outpatient basis
- Performing same-day admission surgery
- Using drug formularies
- Limiting the number of times that insurance will pay for a specific procedure during a set time
- Requiring advance approval for certain procedures and medications
- Requiring referrals as a prerequisite for reimbursing many procedures performed by specialists
- Reviewing charges to determine medical necessity

More aggressive managed care models involve capitation and assumption of financial risk by the practice. Capitation and discounted fee-for-service will be discussed in the section on payment methods. Following are some of the more popular forms of managed care plans:

- **Health maintenance organizations (HMOs):** An HMO is a healthcare system that assumes or shares both the financial risks and the delivery risks associated with providing comprehensive medical services.
- **Preferred provider organizations (PPOs):** A PPO is a medical plan in which coverage is provided to participants through a network of selected healthcare providers (such as hospitals and physicians). The enrollees may go outside the network and pay a greater percentage of the cost of coverage than within the network.

- **Health exchange plans:** Health exchange plans are a mechanism to provide coverage for individuals who do not otherwise have access to coverage. These plans cannot exclude coverage for preexisting conditions and must provide a basic benefit package that includes preventive care as well as catastrophic coverage.
- **Silent PPOs:** Silent PPOs are payers that attempt to obtain discounts similar to contractual allowances without providing a contractual obligation to the provider.

Government and Other Payers

Medicare: Almost all Medicare participants elect Part B coverage. In an attempt to privatize some aspects of Medicare, Medicare Advantage, and Medicare+Choice plans were introduced in 1997. Medicare Advantage plans may be offered in HMO, PPO, private fee-for-service, or special needs plans. The practice and its physicians need to contract separately with these plans. Some of these plans reimburse at Medicare rates, while others have their own fee schedule.

Medicaid: The focus of Medicaid is to cover children and pregnant women living near or below the poverty level.

Other government payers: One such government payer is TRICARE for military healthcare. It was formerly known as the Civilian Health and Medical Program of the Uniformed Services. Another payer is the Civilian Health and Medical Program of the Department of Veterans Affairs.

Workers' Compensation: Most employers must purchase workers' compensation insurance to compensate employees for on-the-job injuries and pay the related medical bills.

Private Pay and Self-Pay: Practices need policies to deal with uninsured patients and uncovered charges for insured patients. Most government and commercial plans include some element of patient responsibility. High-deductible health plans, sometimes combined with health savings accounts (HSAs), are increasing in popularity. HSAs are tax-advantaged savings accounts that allow individuals to set aside money for future medical, retirement, or long-term care premium expenses. Only participants enrolled in a qualified high deductible health plan are eligible for these plans.

Concierge medicine represents a newer form of private pay. Concierge medicine is a private form of practice where doctors charge patients an out-of-pocket retainer fee for full access to their services. Patient loads typically decrease when a physician switches from more traditional fee-per-service practice to concierge medicine.

Third-Party Reimbursement: The bulk of accounts receivable funds received by most practices is from insurance companies and government payers. For accounting purposes, it is important to differentiate between charges (practice fees), allowables (amount to be collected by contract from the insurance company and patient), and paid amount (what the insurance company and patient pays).

Payments come to the practice with an explanation of benefits (EOB). Patient payments are generally in the form of copayments collected at the time of service and deductibles, which are typically billed after insurance payments are collected. Ideally, the combined insurance and patient payment will equal the allowable, which will equal what the contract says should be paid. It is important that the practice knows the contractual allowable to avoid underpayments.

1.4 Revenue Cycle Metrics

A good, computerized practice management system allows the practice to easily produce accounts receivable (A/R) reports. Tracking this data over time, comparing A/R month-to-month or between the current month and the same month from the previous year provides a useful picture of the practice's revenue performance. These snapshots can help the executive understand and anticipate cash flow and spot any potential causes of uncollected debt.

Traditional methods used to control the collection of patient receivables pertains to the following ratios:

1. Gross collection ratio: Collections for the period ÷ gross charges for the period
2. Net collection ratio: Collections for the period ÷ (gross charges — contractual adjustments — charity care for the period)
3. Days in A/R: This ratio indicates how quickly the practice collects its fees or resolves its charges. It is an important indicator in assessing billing and collection performance and is calculated gross accounts receivable/(annual gross charges/365)
4. Accounts receivable turnover: Billings per period (annualized) ÷ average accounts receivable
5. Aging accounts receivable: Percentage of patient accounts in each aging category (typically: 1-30 days, 31-60 days, 61-90 days, 91-120 days and over 120 days)

An aging schedule is an excellent tool to manage patient receivables because it can be integrated with the best control concepts, including management by exception. Improved cash collection will be accomplished by following up with patients who have overdue balances. An automated patient receivables schedule enables financial managers to analyze the performance of one payer versus another.

Monitoring A/R balances month-to-month over time gives a picture of how the practice is doing. Ideally, A/R balances should stay flat or decrease over time. Increases in A/R over time should be investigated. For example, lags in charge posting will contribute to increases in A/R. Processes should be in place to monitor charge posting so that it occurs within 24 hours of payment receipt.

The claim denial rate represents the percentage of claims denied by payers during a given period. This metric quantifies the effectiveness of your revenue cycle management processes. A low denial rate indicates cash flow is healthy, and fewer staff members are needed to maintain that cash flow.[2]

Claim denial rate = total dollar amount of claims denied by payers within a given period/the total dollar amount of claims submitted within the given period

The payer mix is the percentage of revenue coming from private insurance versus government insurance versus self-paying individuals. The mix is important because Medicare and Medicaid often pay less than the cost to treat patients. The percentage is calculated by taking the total payments for a specific payer and dividing it by the total amount of payments for all payers.

Government programs and most private payers use the Resource-Based Relative Value Scale (RBRVS) as the basis for physician payment. The RBRVS assigns relative values to most of the CPT codes. The values are based on the resources that a physician typically uses to perform the service. Because the relative value units (RVUs) summarize the relative weight of the procedures performed by physicians for all patients, regardless of the payer or the physician's charges, executives can use them to evaluate how much an individual physician's activities contribute to practice profits. Executives can also use RVUs to estimate the cost of services provided or determine a physician's compensation.

Total RVUs = total procedures performed by CPT code x RVU (obtained from Medicare RBRVS)

It is important for healthcare executives to become familiar with a variety of metrics, as no single ratio is sufficient to provide a complete picture of the revenue cycle. The executive should become familiar with specialty-specific benchmarks. By using percentages, one can "common size" the metrics so that the practice can be compared to larger or smaller sized practices. Lastly, it is important to utilize internal comparisons to identify trends among payers. Performance dashboards, typically available with practice management systems, can help with this.

1.5 Payer Contracting/Credentialing

The contracting strategy is influenced by the practice plan's organizational structure and business goals as well as the surrounding marketplace. The types of contracts that a medical group will consider will be as diverse as the dynamics of the group itself. Strategies might focus on specific goals of the group practice, for example, primary care growth, network building, affiliated hospital growth, or plan partnership and ownership. In a competitive market, some strategies will focus on maintenance and not growth. Regardless of the specific strategy, educate the medical practice leadership in the specific strategy and measure performance against that strategy.

Despite the myriad opportunities and diverse sources of contracting discussions, there is enormous benefit to centralizing the contract negotiations process. While the contract negotiations process is cleaner and smoother with a central point of contact, that entity should be backed by a committee process that establishes and continuously refines parameters for negotiations. At the onset, this contracting committee will be effective in determining the basics. Items such as the financial threshold for reimbursement (across the group or department by department) and basic business requirements (billing and collecting) should be set by the committee. Over time, however, ensure that the negotiation parameters are further refined. Ultimately, negotiation parameters will correspond in detail to the methods required to effectively operationalize these contracts.

Once a contract concept and the negotiating strategy have been developed, the contract review process should be defined. Every contract requires a thorough review to ensure that practice plan tenets have been met and to ensure that the payer has not introduced unique and potentially unacceptable terms. At a minimum, a checklist should be established and continually refined that will address all the functional requirements of the contract. The signature authority on these contracts should be assured that the contract has met these basic functional requirements as certified by the committee.

Managers of even well-run organizations may not realize they are being underpaid. Several factors contribute to this:

- Many medical groups have complicated systems in place that don't make underpayment obvious
- Various payment arrangements and payment levels, coupled with the volume of managed care contracts, management requirements, and the vast number of transactions complicate the revenue cycle
- Many business offices don't know the actual rate they must collect from a particular health plan for a certain service
- Special payment arrangements in many contracts confuse things further

The result is a constellation of factors that require a sleuth to determine when an underpayment has occurred. The warning signs of contract underperformance, however, are relatively straightforward. The three key warning signs, along with other factors that have led to the development of the provider-payment audit function, are (1) increases in contractual adjustments as a percentage of charges, (2) increases in denials, and (3) increases in days in A/R. It is critical to recognize these high-level warning signs that indicate your organization is losing money it should otherwise be collecting from third-party payers. When you detect one or more signs, launch a detailed payment audit to reveal exactly how much your organization is losing on a payer-by-payer basis. Well-managed provider organizations have come to realize that they can expect to get paid what they negotiated only if they enforce proper payment. The only way to achieve payment compliance is to perform a payer audit. The payer audit function involves a detailed and diligent approach to deciphering complex payment terms. The initial and ongoing investment in this function will substantially pay off: The organization will collect more of its contractually negotiated payments.

Managing Contracts

To create discipline and reinforce consistency, practices can follow a suggested framework, which will improve negotiations and help to effectively manage multiple payer agreements. The five steps are:

1. Preparation
2. Negotiation
3. Implementation
4. Operations
5. Auditing

If there has been a relationship with a payer, preparation should include reviewing the payer's performance. How have they handled denials and appeals? Are their prior authorization expectations realistic or unusually burdensome? Have reimbursements been consistent with the existing contract? Review the current contract and see how the proposed new contract compares, especially in regard to payment and terms of the contract.

If there is no previous relationship with a payer, see what information is available about the payer from other sources. Practices have more leverage with new payers than they realize. A practice may be wise to refuse an evergreen clause until the insurance company proves itself.[3]

To ensure contract compliance, contract language must be thoroughly reviewed, and potentially negotiated. Areas of risk in contracts are:

- Identification of covered products
- Medical necessity — who makes clinical decisions?
- Indemnification
- Claims payment — as determined by federal and state laws
- Provider manual — operational details of contract are here
- Termination and renewal
- Access to records, including financial records
- Appeals and denials
- Compensation — details around payment
- Governing law

Operationalizing contracts takes far more energy than the contract negotiations themselves. In fact, operationalizing contracts will ensure the success of a contract as much as or more so than the negotiation process. Like the contracting committee, a managed care team should be formed to address contract implementation. The team should have representation from the following functional areas: patient accounting, information systems, contract and financial analysis, clinical operations, and medical management. Ideally, if these functions occur within affiliate hospitals, representatives should be recruited to join the managed care team.

As with the contracting committee, a checklist should be developed representing all aspects of contract implementation. The checklist for fee-for-service agreements includes the following functional requirements: admitting and ambulatory care, billing and collections, contract management, financial review and analysis, staff and physician education, information systems, medical management, reporting, credentialing, and directories. A more expansive checklist would be required for capitation agreements, to include risk management structures, auditing functions, carve-out management and auditing, medical management, physician payment and incentives, as well as financial analysis. Additionally, if the financial value of the contract merits the resource, it is important to consider designating an operations leader as the liaison for the agreement.

Practices may be concerned about the added cost of a designated staff member to manage contracts. Often, this resource will pay for itself in terms of maximizing reimbursement from the payer and holding the payer accountable to the fundamental terms of the contract itself. Bear in mind, this resource does add overhead costs. Contract value and the size of the relationship are key to determining whether this resource is warranted and can have influence.[4]

Developing Negotiation Skills

Effectively negotiating contracts is both an art and a science. The following recommendations are helpful during the negotiation process:

- Be prepared with data
- Meet face-to-face if possible
- Be aware of your negotiating style and how it is seen by the other party
- Stay focused on your objectives and goals
- Define the deal breakers
- Be professional
- Be inventive
- Persevere

Establishing Personal Contacts with Each Major Carrier

While payer partnerships are elusive, the contracting and implementation process should set the expectation of a payer partnership. Contracts should stipulate mandatory meetings and specify requirements for data transfer, including the scope and timing of transfers. Setting expectations via the practice plan will create greater accountability by the payer and assist in forging partnerships through the term of the relationship. Performance measurements should be considered as well. Learning the payer's systems, in general terms, will assist in problem resolution throughout the contract. While payers and providers don't have consistent goals regarding payment for clinical services, there is still some efficiency and improved workflow created by forging stronger partnerships.[5]

Credentialing

CAQH Credentialing refers to the process of self-reporting demographic, education and training, work history, malpractice history, National Provider Identifier numbers, continuing education and other relevant credentialing information to create an online profile for insurance companies to access.

The practice will generally need to submit this information in connection with the initial contract, and periodically thereafter, usually every one to three years. The practice usually needs to provide similar information when applying for or renewing hospital privileges or malpractice insurance. The practice should designate an individual responsible for credentialing.

Getting new providers credentialed on a timely basis is important. The practice cannot generally get paid for new providers' services until those forms are completed, processed, and approved. This is part of the administrative workload involved in adding a new physician to the practice. Credentialing a new physician normally takes from one to five months, or even longer, depending on the carrier, the time of year, and whether the physician is new to the state. Credentialing can take longer in the summer and around the holiday season, when the credentialing committees do not meet as frequently. This process may also take longer when the practice is hiring a physician from another state.

1.6 Revenue Cycle Regulations

The healthcare executive must be familiar with national and state regulations as they relate to the medical practice billing. The Centers for Medicare and Medicaid Services (CMS) administers the Medicare and Medicaid programs that provide health insurance coverage.

CMS plays a significant role in the regulatory oversight of physicians and other providers because many physicians accept Medicare beneficiaries and rely on those medical revenues. Because of the size of its insured population, the agency's rules and payment policies often set the tone for the policies of private insurance companies. Violating these rules can result in fines, civil or criminal actions, and temporary or permanent expulsion from participating in Medicare and Medicaid programs.

The insurance commissioner is a public official in the executive branch of a state who regulates the insurance industry for the state in which they hold office. Healthcare executives need to be familiar with state laws including recoupment laws, surprise billing laws, and prompt payment legislation.

1.7 In-House Billing vs. Outsourcing

Some practices outsource billing services to a third party to gain control over billing problems and increase revenue. Other practices feel that keeping those services in-house is safer and more cost-effective. In-house billing is generally more cost-effective in smaller practices, where practices are better able to control their office's productivity. Problems can be addressed more quickly when billing is performed in-house, since the billing staff is located in the same office as the physician and other caregivers. They can improve efficiency more easily since workers are directly employed by the office. Time isn't wasted contacting the right person at the outsourcing company and waiting for a response. Direct communication between billers and providers means that the billing staff can receive rapid responses to questions on medical coding and patient information.

Practices find outsourcing billing initially more expensive than in-house billing, although it can save money in the long run. The return on investment (ROI) for outsourcing generally becomes greater as the size of the practice increases. Companies that specialize in medical billing typically have greater expertise and resources in this area than a medical practice. They can also provide a practice with software solutions such as billing and practice management. The cost of maintaining trained billing staff is moved to the outsourced company, and the companies generally charge a percentage of the practice's revenue, thereby relieving the administrative burden of an in-house billing team. For more information, review Patrick Dougherty's "Pros and Cons of Outsourcing Medical Billing."[6]

Most billing arrangements involve some work in-house, even if billing is outsourced. Oversight is still of paramount importance and should include regular meetings and review of revenue cycle metrics. When considering making a transition, it is important for the healthcare executive to consider all relevant costs in the comparison including changes to cash flow during the transition.

1.8 Billing/Coding Audits

The complexity of coding and documenting professional services makes mistakes likely. Providers may miscode services at a higher or lower level or fail to provide enough documentation to justify the code selected. Downcoding, which is entering a lower-than-appropriate code, causes lower reimbursements and skews measurements of provider productivity. Coding at a higher-than-justified level, or upcoding, can lead payers to suspect fraud. The repercussions can include payer audits of the practice's records, or worse, civil or criminal charges against the provider and possible suspension or exclusion from the payer's program. Therefore, it is critical that executives implement a program of compliance with federal billing and coding requirements. The Office of Inspector General for Health and Human Services, which has the authority to exclude providers from the Medicare and Medicaid programs, recommends that a practice routinely review bills and medical notes for compliance with coding, billing, and documentation requirements. Keep in mind that both downcoding and upcoding can be found to be fraudulent and or abusive. Some providers might undercode to reduce deductible costs with intent to save money for the patient, for example.

When initiating a compliance program, the practice must determine whether to review claims retrospectively or concurrently, as they are submitted. The auditing system can begin with a baseline audit, only examining claims submitted during the three-month period immediately after the compliance program begins. Follow-up audits should be conducted at least annually to ensure that the practice's compliance program is being followed.

Types of Auditors

There are three types of auditors generally involved in the various audit examinations: independent (external), internal, and government auditors:

- Independent (External) Auditors: The audits of financial statements are performed by independent accountants, usually CPAs. Independent CPAs do not hold an ownership interest or have management involvement in the clients they audit, and therefore lend the utmost credibility to their work.
- Internal Auditors: Unlike independent auditors, internal auditors are employed within the organization and only perform services for that firm. Internal auditors conduct operational and compliance audits for their employer. Their role is to determine whether the organization and its employees are complying with established policies and procedures. They usually report to the governing body or to some committee of the board of directors. As medical groups grow in size and scope of operations, groups will employ internal auditors to conduct compliance audits and reviews.
- Government auditors: Government auditors conduct audits under the auspices of various governmental agencies, such as the General Accounting Office and the IRS. They usually perform compliance audits to evaluate whether federal laws and regulations are being followed.
- Payers including Medicare and Medicaid, and commercial insurers may also conduct audits. Medicare Recovery Audit Programs (or RAC) are routinely conducted by private contractors on behalf of Medicare to assure proper payment.

1.9 Segregation of Duties in the Revenue Cycle

An effective internal control process requires that cash functions be divided among personnel in such a manner that makes embezzlement, mishandling and theft of cash more difficult. This means that employees with cash functions should not perform multiple functions, so responsibilities for handling cash, recording transactions, and authorizing transactions should be separated. No one person should have complete authority over the entire sequence of transactions that involve cash (e.g., from the purchase of a resource through payment).

Smaller offices sometimes have difficulty achieving good separation of duties. A practice can often achieve appropriate segregation of duties by expanding some responsibilities beyond the core administrative staff. The practice might use non-administrative staff or outside accountants to perform certain functions. For cash, the two primary areas requiring segregation of duties are (1) cash receipts and (2) cash disbursements. Make sure that those employees who receive cash receipts are not allowed access to the payment posting and adjustment functions. Maximize use of bank lockboxes and electronic payments to minimize the amount of cash that is physically in the office. This enhances segregation of duties by preventing office staff from having access to that cash.

Common types of revenue cycle fraud include the following:

- Skimming: The perpetrator simply takes the money before it is recorded on the organization's books. The perpetrator may either skim revenue, supplies, or assets.
- Lapping: The name for a receivables skimming scheme where an embezzler misappropriates a payment from Patient A, posts a payment from Patient B to Patient A's account, posts a payment from Patient C to Patient B's account, and so forth, until the perpetrator pays back all the patients' accounts, the scheme is uncovered, or another form of fraud is used to cover the embezzler's tracks.
- Cash larceny: This is stealing incoming cash after it has been recorded on the books, which often involves destroying or falsifying records.

SAMPLE QUESTIONS

1. Examples of front-end revenue cycle activities include all of the following except:

A. Charge capture and charge entry

B. Billing and claims production

C. Appointment scheduling

D. Patient registration and insurance verification

2. Which is a valuable indicator of the efficiency and speed of your billing and collection activities?

A. Total accounts receivable

B. Days in accounts receivable

C. Overhead percentage

D. Bad debt ratio

3. Some of the variables that should be tracked on payers are accuracy of claims payment, timeliness of payments, number of denials, resolution of appeals, and:

A. Audits

B. Contract renewal frequency

C. Contract negotiations

D. Coordination of benefits

Answers: 1-B, 2-B, 3-C

TASK 2: CASH FLOW MANAGEMENT

KEY TERMS

Float: The lag period from when a check is issued to the time when the check clears the issuer's checking account.

Compensating balances: Additional requirements imposed on borrowers by commercial banks beyond interest charges and requiring the borrower to maintain a specified demand deposit balance at that bank. Inadequate compensating balances may result in additional service charges, difficulty in obtaining loans, or higher interest rates.

2.1 Monitoring Bank Balance

Some groups may desire only the information on account balances. In addition to book (or checkbook) balances, bank balances may be obtained using Internet or telephone banking. This information serves at least two purposes: (1) determining the float position of each account and (2) determining the adequacy of compensating balances.

Groups that do not maintain a cash budget or short-term cash plan might want to use a cash forecast for the next few days. Financial managers are strongly encouraged to use daily cash reports because they improve cash planning by helping to avert cash crises and allowing a more even distribution of cash to physicians.

Using daily cash forecasts will frequently lead to a lower financing cost for operations, a stronger credit standing, and more satisfied physicians. The healthcare executive may find it useful to keep a month-to-date cash spreadsheet, which details the receipts, disbursements, transfers, and running balance by bank account by day for each month.

2.2 Projecting Cash Flows

For most medical groups, cash flow projections by day for the next week, and then by week for the remainder of the month, provide an adequate approach to managing short-term cash. For example, the short-term cash plan presents four weeks of data showing daily cash flows for week one and weekly cash flows for weeks two, three, and four. At the end of each week, the short-term cash plan is rolled over. A new short-term cash plan will show on a daily basis the expected cash flows for week 2 and show on a weekly basis the expected cash flows for weeks three, four, and five. This arrangement will continually roll over each week, thereby keeping the short-term cash plan current.

Fluctuations in cash flow are very much a part of doing business as a medical group. When special expenses are added on top of the normal cash flow ups and downs, the probabilities of an occasional monthly shortfall increase dramatically.

Making sure that the medical group has an adequate base of working capital (usually short-term lines of credit from commercial banks) is one way to guard against these circumstances.

2.3 Bank Reconciliation

Bank reconciliations need to be performed by a person who does not have responsibility for cash or maintaining the related accounting records. In the past, good internal control practices included promptly performing reconciliations on a monthly basis upon receiving bank statements in the mail at the beginning of the month. With the advent of Internet banking, practices can reconcile bank balances at any time during the month. Moreover, today's increased frequency of electronic transactions, including both cash receipts and disbursements, makes more frequent review of bank activity and bank reconciliations a recommended practice. No matter the frequency of the reconciliations, any discrepancies need to be reported immediately and investigated. Depending on the findings, changes in policies and procedures, employee assignments and new controls may be needed to assure that problems are contained, and no future issues will arise. The degree of the issue may require reporting to senior management, physician owner, or key stakeholders.

Practices should view their bank account activity online on an ongoing basis and reconcile their bank balance on an interim basis throughout the month. The increased potential for fraud demands that the practice be vigilant in reviewing this data. Unauthorized or questionable transactions should be reported promptly to the bank, as the time frame for reporting these items and being reimbursed for the related losses may be short. Also, banks may consider a lack of certain internal controls within the practice a sufficient reason for not reimbursing those losses. In connection with the setup and ongoing use of its Internet banking function, the practice should be vigilant about internet security. Be careful about who has access to view bank account information and even more vigilant about who is given authority to initiate and authorize funds transactions.

2.4 Petty Cash Reconciliation

Petty cash should be available to take care of minor incidentals for the practice. Internal controls are necessary to assure that the fund is used appropriately, including monthly reconciliation, and requiring paper receipts to keep a paper trail of all transactions. Cash should be replenished once the amount dips below a predetermined level, and petty cash should be kept separate from any patient receipts.

2.5 Cash Receipt Process

Specific individuals — and only those people — should be designated to handle and be responsible for cash. Furthermore, the practice should segregate the functions relating to cash receipts to ensure that the individuals who handle cash and checks do not post the payments and related adjustments, and still another individual performs the bank reconciliation.

Accounting records must be kept by those who do not handle or have access to cash. Front office staff should not be permitted to record transactions in patient accounts receivable, and accountants responsible for receivables should not physically handle cash receipts or payment.

Finally, still another person should be responsible for reconciling the bank account. This person should not handle cash or post the accounting records. All cash receipts should be deposited intact daily. No payments should be made out of undeposited cash receipts. Only the petty cash or change fund should remain on the premises overnight. A verifiable record should be made immediately after each cash receipt, such as a remittance advice.

Tips for managing control over cash receipts:

- Medical billing software generally allows for assigning staff members access to different functions. Make sure that those employees who receive cash receipts are not allowed access to the payment posting and adjustment functions.
- Maximize use of bank lockboxes and electronic payments to minimize the amount of cash that is physically in the office. This enhances segregation of duties by avoiding office staff access to that cash.
- If your practice receives checks from patients and insurance companies in the mail, consider having two staff members open the mail together.
- Use a check-scanning machine at the office that transmits the check information to the bank for electronic deposit. To further eliminate the potential for embezzlement or misplacement of checks, have the checkout personnel scan the check in front of patients and give them their receipts at that time.
- Centralize cash receipts whenever possible.
- Receipts should be issued anytime cash is received, using a pre-numbered receipt book.
- Conduct unannounced cash counts.
- All cash receipts should be deposited intact daily.
- Cash receipts should be reconciled daily, with appropriate documentation (cash reports, receipt books, etc.). No payments should be made out of undeposited cash receipts.

2.6 Segregation of Duties Over Cash Flow

The practice should also ensure proper segregation of duties among employees with cash disbursement functions. Authorizing disbursements, preparing checks, maintaining the A/P records, signing checks, and mailing or distributing checks should all be performed by different individuals. Yet another person with no other cash disbursement responsibilities should reconcile the bank account.

In some smaller practices, the functions of signing checks and authorizing transactions are combined. While it is important for the check signer to review the supporting documentation for all of the checks that they sign, it is especially important for check signers who bear the sole responsibility for authorizing transactions.

Medical groups should also use the following internal controls related to cash disbursements:

- Cash disbursements should be made by check or by bank ACH, unless specifically authorized from petty cash.
- The checks should be prenumbered, and the stock of blank checks should be kept under adequate safeguards with access given only to persons authorized to sign checks.
- Voided checks should be destroyed. If the group prefers to save these, then it should (1) tear out the signature portion of the check and (2) keep them under safeguards similar to blank checks.
- No payments should be made without proper authorization and verification of the amounts due. When checks are signed, the signer should have all supporting documentation available for review to ensure that the disbursements are valid and appropriate. Some practices may consider dual signatures on their checks, but with proper controls this may be unnecessary.

Additional recommendations for segregation of cash flow:

- Limit employee IT access only to those areas they need.
- Require authorization of purchases, payroll, and disbursements.
- Separate handling receipts and deposits from recordkeeping functions (recording transactions and reconciling accounts).
- Separate purchasing functions from payables functions.
- Ensure the same person isn't authorized to write and sign a check.
- When opening mail, endorse or stamp checks "for deposit only" and list checks on a log before turning them over to the person responsible for depositing receipts. Periodically reconcile the incoming check log against the deposit.
- Require supervisors to approve employee time sheets before payroll is prepared.
- If the agency is so small that you can't separate duties, require an independent check of work being done, for example, by a board member.
- Require accounting department employees to take vacations so that records can be assessed for any fraudulent activity.

The suggested segregation of duties over cash receipts is shown in Exhibit 2.1.[7]

EXHIBIT 2.1
Segregation of Duties for Cash Receipts

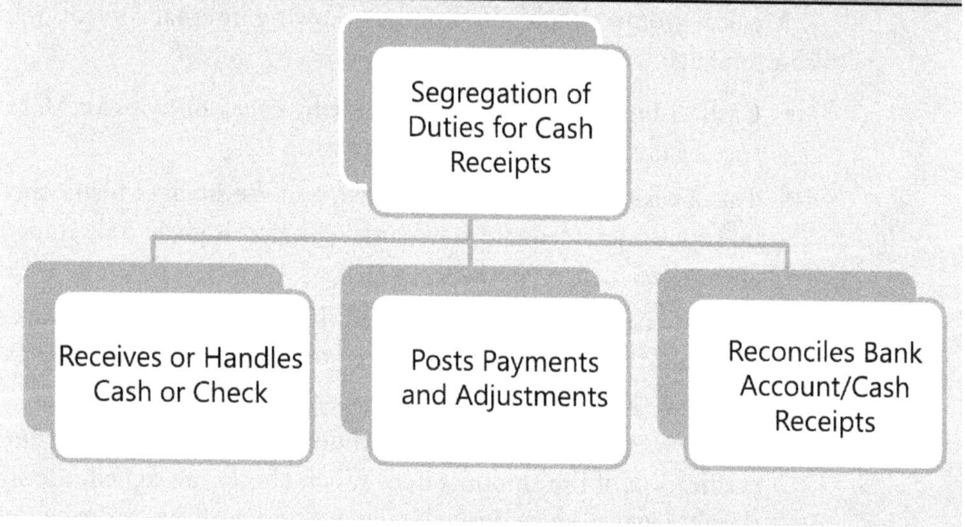

SAMPLE QUESTIONS

1. Which most accurately describes a short-term cash plan?

A. A list of targeted collections from patients at time of service

B. A plan that anticipates cash collections and disbursements over the next four weeks on a rolling basis

C. A financial statement that is a major component of the practice's external financial reporting

D. A summary of cash collections and disbursements for the previous month

2. What is the primary purpose of developing a policy on internal control of cash receipts?

A. To provide a secure place for storage of cash and checks

B. To reduce errors in bank reconciliation

C. To ensure that patient payments are deposited daily

D. To protect cash collections from theft or fraud

3. Which step reduces the risk of fraud and embezzlement?

A. Requiring each employee to take time away from the office

B. Advising patients to make checks payable to the physician, not the practice

C. Requiring one trustworthy employee to control the entire sequence of cash transactions

D. Requiring employees with the authority to sign checks to also make bank deposits

Answers: 1-B, 2-D, 3-A

TASK 3: ACCOUNTS PAYABLE MANAGEMENT

Payment of bills is popularly known as *accounts payable*, or A/P. Management of A/P requires knowledge of basic bookkeeping, accounting software, standard vendor payment processes, and internal cash controls in order to support an effective practice financial infrastructure.

KEY TERMS

Accounting system: Organized set of manual and computerized accounting methods, procedures, and controls established to gather, record, classify, analyze, summarize, interpret, and present accurate and timely financial data for management decisions.

Segregation of duties: Separation of duties or responsibilities to prevent fraud and errors. Divide the tasks and associated privileges for a specific business process among multiple users. The traditional example of segregation of duties is the requirement that the person who receives cash receipts not be the person who records cash receipts and adjustments.

3.1 Basic Bookkeeping

Healthcare executives should understand the basic financial statements that the practice needs to maintain on a regular basis. These include the:

- Balance sheet
- Income statement
- Statement of changes in equity
- Statement of cash flows

These financial statements may be prepared using the accrual basis of accounting in accordance with generally accepted accounting principles or some other comprehensive basis of accounting, such as the cash or tax basis.

All business and public entities have legal requirements to maintain accurate and representative accounting records that accurately show the financial status of the organization. Likewise, all businesses and public entities need reliable, relevant, and consistent accounting information for managerial decision-making.

Whether an organization is a public entity or a private business, it needs to record its financial condition. The chart of accounts lists the accounts that are used to record the organization's expenses and revenues, as well as its assets and liabilities. The chart of accounts defines the level of detail that the organization's accounting system will record and also provides the vocabulary of the accounting system.

Accounts Payable Cycle

A/P are amounts owed to vendors and suppliers for goods and services acquired on a credit basis and for which the suppliers have not yet been paid. Usually, these claims are unsecured and are frequently referred to as *open accounts*. The terms of these payable transactions normally require payment within 10 to 60 days after receipt of the goods or services.

When the practice receives goods or services, the invoice should be recorded in the A/P accounting system. The chart of accounts should have sufficient detail around the different types of goods and services so that management can adequately track utilization and budget appropriately. At the same time, the invoice should be compared with the purchase order or contract and actual materials received to verify the accuracy of the invoice. Processing A/P includes maintaining a detailed record of individual accounts by vendor and using a system to identify dates on which the obligations should be paid.

The terms of these transactions sometimes allow cash discounts, such as 2/10 net 30. (That is, if the invoice is paid within 10 days from the date of the invoice, the payer can take a 2% discount from the amount due. If the discount is not taken, then the total amount due is to be paid by 30 days from the date of the invoice.) Missing cash discounts can be costly; thus, the system should ensure that all cash discounts are taken when available. Here are three strategies for effective management of vendor accounts:

1. Ask suppliers to bill the medical group for all purchases on a set series of dates each month to prevent payments from bunching up and to ease the demands on cash outflows.
2. Find out if vendors will grant a larger discount for paying cash at the time of purchase rather than being billed later. Sometimes discounts up to 5% are possible.
3. Practice should monitor timeliness of invoice payment.

Once the invoice has been paid it should be marked as such. Each month management and the board should be aware of what's been paid, and any irregularities found such as discounts not taken.

Some goods, such as printer paper, must be generally available; others, such as pharmaceuticals, should be accessible only to appropriate staff, with limited access. In addition, the practice should track inventory periodically against utilization to assure theft is not occurring. Those practices with significant inventory should consider the use of inventory software.

Obtain Payment Approvals and Receipt of Delivery

Documentation of the purchase of goods and services, including purchase authorizations, receiving slips, and vendor invoices, along with independent verification of the transaction by examining these documents, needs to occur before payment is made. The functions of authorizing disbursements, preparing checks, maintaining the A/P records, signing checks, and mailing or distributing checks should be performed by different individuals.

No payments should be made without proper authorization and verification of the amounts due. When checks are signed, the signer should have all supporting documentation available for review to ensure that the disbursements are valid and appropriate.

Incoming orders should always be checked against order slips and packing slips for accuracy and completeness, and invoices and vendor bills should be reconciled to these documents.

General Accounting

Accounting software comes in a variety of shapes and sizes. The following is a breakdown of some of the more common features accounting software offers:

- Accounts payable: Applications handling accounts payable (A/P) functions help automate recording the liabilities and paying the bills that the practice receives from vendors for purchases it makes. You can use A/P software to schedule payments and issue checks to vendors.
- General ledger: The general ledger application is the primary focus of many accounting software packages. The general ledger contains the details for the activity in each of the accounts in the chart of accounts. It collects information the practice needs to prepare its financial statements and tax returns. It is an important source of data for internal analyses, including cost analyses.
- Accounts receivable: In the A/R application you can automatically track outstanding invoices for collection and payment. Most A/R applications provide reports to help track payments before they become outdated. Medical practices often manage their A/R in their practice management software rather than directly in their accounting software. The information from the practice management software or billing company will often flow to the accounting software's general ledger via an interface or other connection or by journal entry.
- Payroll: Payroll applications often coincide with accounting software to enable businesses to keep track of employee pay rates, taxes, deductions, and even accrued or used vacation hours. You can usually generate W-2 forms and other important documents using payroll applications. Some payroll applications allow for storing of human resource data.
- Budgeting and forecasting: Applications handling budgeting and forecasting help you track your financial performance against your expected budget throughout the year. Look for a program with a planning module to help you plan your finances for the year.

Track the Flow of Financial Information

Accounting systems take the cash and accruals from various transactions and generate financial reports and statements (See Exhibit 2.2).

EXHIBIT 2.2

Data Flow Within a Medical Group Accounting System

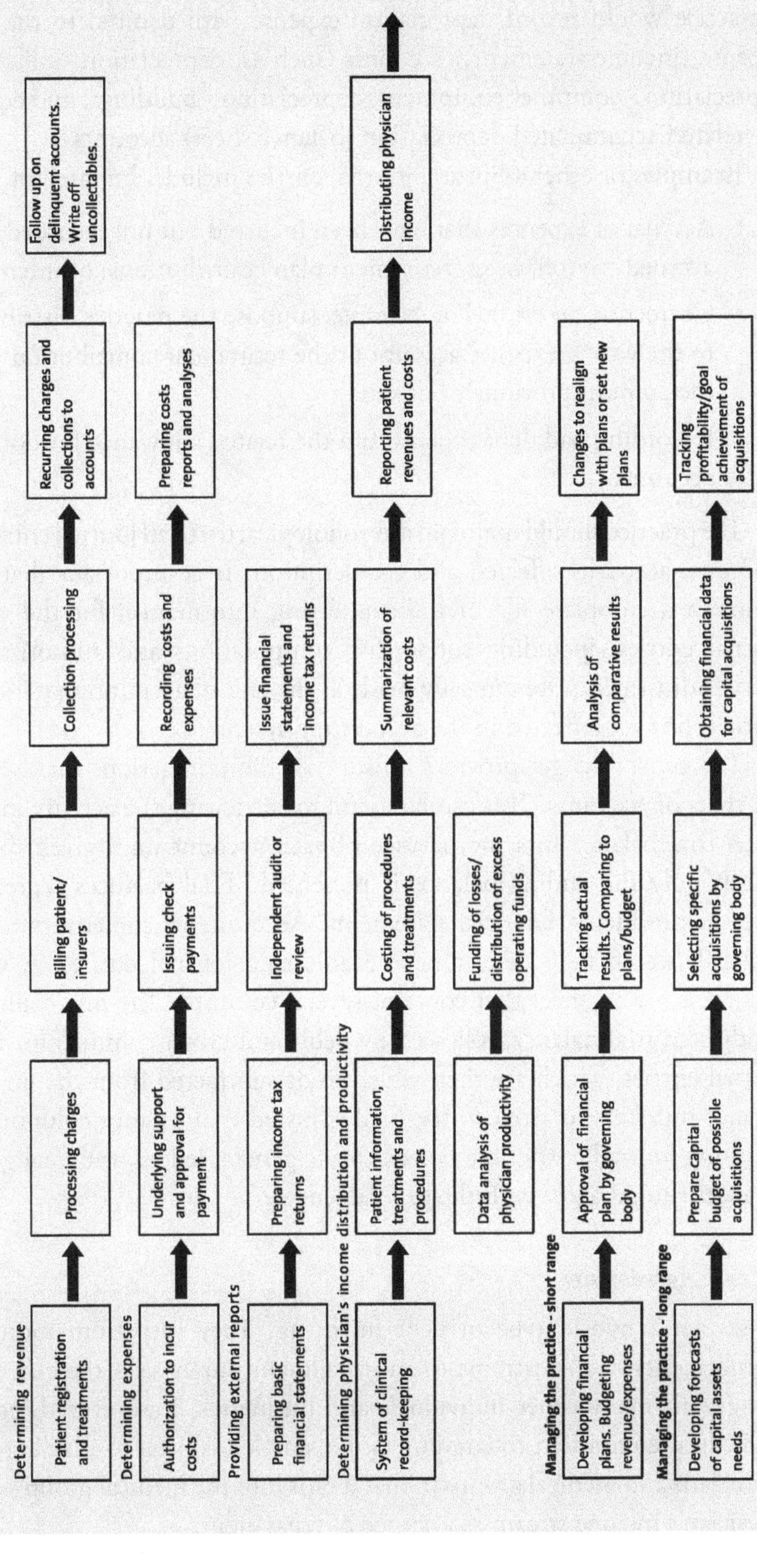

The first step is to create adjusting journal entries to record transactions, such as depreciation, which have not yet been recorded, but are necessary for the financial statements to be correct. Each transaction must have an equal number of debits and credits, so that the accounting system will remain in balance. For example, a practice would record depreciation expense with debit(s) to the depreciation expense (income statements) accounts (such as: depreciation - office equipment, depreciation - computer equipment, depreciation - buildings) and equal credits to the related accumulated depreciation (balance sheet) accounts.

Examples of other adjusting journal entries include, but are not limited to:

- Accrual of expenses that have been incurred but not recorded, such as accrued payroll, taxes, retirement plan contributions, or interest.
- Correcting an error. For example, suppose the practice distributed a check to the wrong expense account or the retirement contribution is less than the amount previously booked.
- Recording bad debt expense and the related allowance for doubtful accounts.

The practice should maintain a chronological list of all journal entries, including amounts, accounts affected and a description. It is important that the practice maintain a complete file of the supporting information for the computerized journal entries, including supporting computations and authorization for the entry. Adjustments are typically made at the end of accounting periods to record accruals not yet reflected in the accounting system.

The general ledger provides a listing of the transactions for each account in the chart of accounts. This can be useful for reviewing the activity in an account.

A trial balance lists the balance of each account on a given date. Unlike a ledger, only the ending balance is presented. Trial balances represent the first piece in producing financial statements. Accountants sometimes use a working trial balance to help determine the adjusting journal entries. A working trial balance is a worksheet that contains several columns. The first column is for the unadjusted trial balance, followed by debit and credit columns for the adjusting journal entries, which are then added to or subtracted from the unadjusted trial balance numbers to arrive at the final adjusted trial balance column(s). After the adjusting journal entries are posted to the general ledger, the final general ledger balances should agree with the general ledger.

Understand Lease Agreements

Leases are a hybrid type of debt financing. They vary from month-to-month arrangements at one extreme to an installment purchase at the other. Physicians, along with many other individuals and businesses, lease everything from autos to medical equipment to computers. Leasing lends itself to funding the needs of physicians and medical groups in that it taps into the medical group's or individual physician's income stream as a source of repayment.

When it comes to high-tech equipment and computers, many physicians prefer leasing because it limits maintenance and repair headaches and reduces the chances of being stuck with equipment that is technologically obsolete. Leasing is a useful component of most financing structures. However, given the magnitude of aggressive medical groups' capital needs, it is usually a small part of the total financing picture. Also, financial managers should be concerned with the large number of physicians and other individuals who do not view leases as debt, and as a result, are often lulled into a false sense of financial security.

Types of leases vary. Most automobile companies or equipment manufacturers or distributors will offer leasing programs to physicians and medical groups. These offers need a careful analysis of the full cost versus borrowing the money or paying for the equipment from the practice's cash flow. In other words, leasing may not be as good as it sounds. Two of the most commonly available lease arrangements are *operating leases* and *financing leases*. Operating leases (a true lease) are rental agreements that typically have a shorter term than the useful economic life of the asset leased, with ownership remaining with the lessor at the end of the lease. Operating leases usually involve office space, automobiles, or office furniture. Finance (capital) leases frequently cover periods that approximate the useful economic life of the item being leased. They are typically for a longer term than operating leases and may include a purchase option that would allow the lessee to gain ownership of the asset over the life of the lease.

3.2 Segregation of Duties and Other Internal Controls

When assessing internal controls, management should have a clear, well-defined strategy. This strategy should include specific documentation, audits, and verifiable results that permit someone not connected with the process to understand the procedure and verify the outcome through the internal control system.

Preventing unauthorized access to the practice's assets is the primary goal of internal controls in regard to cash management. Ensuring that cash on hand is reconciled, accounted for, and compared with actual amounts should be accomplished daily. Internal controls should cover items such as the protection of unauthorized access to prenumbered checks or receipts. All fees collected at the time of service should be accounted for. The use of a bank lockbox is another crucial internal control.

Establishing a system for the authorization of purchases, competitive bidding, and verification of the receipt of purchased items is critical. While a compliance program will cover many areas of internal controls within transaction management, other areas also need close scrutiny. A healthcare executive should ask if internal controls are in place to capture proper coding and payment posting. Contract negotiation, establishing fee schedules, capturing lost revenues through claim denials, refund approvals with supporting documentation, and so forth, are all areas that need multiple internal controls to assist in billing and capturing revenue.

Specific individuals in the group should be designated to handle and be responsible for cash. Others should not be permitted to do so. Furthermore, the practice should segregate the functions relating to cash receipts to ensure that the person(s) who handles cash and checks does not post the payments and related adjustments, and still another person performs the bank reconciliation. Accounting records must be kept by persons who do not handle or have access to cash. Thus, cashiers should not be permitted to record transactions in patient A/R, and accountants responsible for receivables should not physically handle cash receipts or payment. Finally, still another person should be responsible for reconciling the bank account. This person should not handle cash or post the accounting records.

SAMPLE QUESTION

1. **Matching invoices to be paid with packing slips is part of what process?**

   A. Accounts payable

   B. Cash reconciliation

   C. Cash accounting

   D. Amortization

Answer: 1-A

TASK 4: PAYROLL MANAGEMENT

4.1 Payroll Lifecycle

Key skills related to payroll management include establishing policies and procedures, overseeing the reporting system to capture work hours, comparing benchmarks, reporting taxes, and establishing guidelines for the payroll deduction process. Although many practices employ external organizations to implement payroll processing and reporting, it is essential for any healthcare executive to understand the overall flow, regulatory requirements, and functions of a high-performing payroll system.

The payroll process has three main steps:

1. Paying the employee
2. Paying employer portion of payroll taxes and transferring employee-deducted taxes to relevant government authorities
3. Filing tax reporting forms with relevant government authorities

A practice must decide on these elements to manage and process payroll:

- Payment frequency
  - Bi-weekly or another basis
  - The day of the week on which payment is made
  - How it is distributed (e.g. check versus electronic deposit)
- Job functions and pay ranges
  - Employees should be paid in accordance with their exempt/nonexempt status
  - Each position should have a pay range with minimums and maximums
- Time recording
  - Most practices use an automated/online time and attendance system
  - The practice should have clear policies on how they treat breaks, mealtime, and time off, and inform employees regarding those policies
- Overtime and bonus policies
  - Payment of any overtime or shift differentials and required approvals
  - Qualifications for and timing of bonuses (performance and holiday)
  - Use of bonuses for employees who have "topped out"
- Clear communication on payroll deductions
  - Taxes
  - Employee insurance plans
  - Retirement plan, 401(b), 401(k) or 403(b) contributions
  - Donations or contributions to community organizations
  - Mandated deductions, such as garnishments, child support, or tax levies

Processing Payroll

The practice should have a formal process by which staff members can report hours worked and/or hours off for each pay period. Typically, the pay period will be recorded in two-week increments with 40 hours per week.

The payroll reporting system should:

- Record time off for vacations, sick leave, meetings, jury duty, and/or bereavement
- Reflect the practice's policies and procedures relating the matrix of different types of paid time off, time accrued in each category, and the past cycle's hours utilized and paid
- Create reports for tracking and identifying hours worked and time off by each individual
- Calculate and report pension deferrals and benefits contributions and report the remaining taxable income accurately
- Calculate and report taxes paid by the practice
- Calculate and report taxes withheld from the employee
- Generate end-of-year tax documents for employees and the practice

At the conclusion of a payroll cycle, the employees' supervisor should approve each timecard including overtime hours. Human resources should notify the person responsible for payroll of any changes in employee status (pay rates, withholdings, benefits, termination) along with the date the change is effective.

Payroll can be distributed via check or direct deposit. Direct deposit is the cleanest way to distribute pay. At the same time, employees need documentation of the gross and net pay along with deductions for benefits, taxes and withholdings for the current period and year-to-date. This can be handled by distribution of a check stub or by access to a payroll portal where employees can sign in to view their payroll information.

When a new payroll system is installed or when there are updates to the current system, management should do a test to assure accuracy. One of the most critical management responsibilities is to assure there are no payroll errors.

Payroll Methods

The process of payroll can occur using one of three methods:

1. The practice prepares the employees' payroll internally
2. The practice hires a certified public accountant (CPA) and/or bookkeeper to process the payroll checks
3. The practice outsources payroll to a payroll vendor

Payroll reports should be reviewed at least each payroll cycle.

Processing payroll internally usually requires the purchase of software with this capability. Many smaller practices use this option, although it can be risky if the practice does not have a staff member who is proficient in payroll requirements.

If you hire a CPA or bookkeeper to process payroll, you must ensure that the person performing the duties is, in fact, experienced and knowledgeable.

Outsourcing payroll has become more popular in the past few years as the tax laws have become more complicated. However, outsourcing firms may not be able to readily provide data in the format that you request, unless it offers a flexible design. For instance, each type of paid hour, such as regular, overtime, and time off, i.e., jury duty, vacation, and bereavement, should have a unique designation for input and reporting. It may also be more difficult to communicate your needs easily with a large firm.

New Hires

Preferably before, but certainly on their first day, new employees need to go through a process to assure accurate and timely payment and payroll. These steps include:

- Completion of the federal W-4 tax withholding form
- State and city withholding tax forms
- Employee benefit enrollment forms
- Any other information

In addition, procedures for time reporting should be reviewed with the employee along with an explanation of all benefits.

4.2 Employment and Payroll Regulatory Requirements

Financial managers should obtain copies of relevant payroll-related laws and regulations, and may want to subscribe to a payroll information service to gain access to an ongoing stream of updated information. Some of the related payroll areas that financial managers should gain familiarity with include:

- Federal wage and hour requirements, including:
  - Exempt and nonexempt employees
  - Minimum wage requirements
  - Overtime pay
  - Employer records
  - Breaks
  - Employee versus independent contractor status determination
  - Workers with disabilities
  - Termination
  - Leaves of absence
- Discrimination, including:
  - Federal legislation (e.g., Civil Rights Act) regarding prohibited actions, sexual harassment, and employer obligations
  - Age discrimination

  - Disability accommodations and discrimination
  - Affirmative action
  - National Labor Relations Board provisions regarding prohibited practices and penalties
- Payroll requirements, including:
  - Federal and state income tax
  - Federal Insurance Contributions Act (FICA) tax
  - Deposit of payroll taxes
  - Federal (FUTA) and state (SUTA) unemployment taxes
  - Federal and state tax returns
  - Workers' compensation regulations and requirements
- Employee deferrals and deductions relating to benefits, such as:
  - Health insurance
  - 401(k) plans
  - Short and long-term disability insurance
  - Flexible and dependent spending accounts
- Post-employment issues
  - Consolidated Omnibus Budget Reconciliation Act of 1985 (COBRA) qualifications and payments

4.3 Payroll Liabilities

Payroll is a type of accounts payable. The employer pays employees' wages after withholding the employees' portion of payroll taxes. The employer then calculates its own portion of payroll taxes and transfers employee and employer taxes to appropriate taxing authorities. Some tax considerations include:

- **Federal withholding taxes:** These are determined from the required W-4 form completed by all new employees.
- **Social Security:** Also known as FICA or OASDI (Old-Age, Survivors, and Disability Insurance). The current employee tax rate and wage base (maximum wage limit) can be found on the Social Security Administration website. The employer is required to match the employee's contribution.
- **Medicare:** As of 2020, both the employee and the employer are taxed at a rate of 1.45% each. The Patient Protection and Affordable Care Act established a new additional Medicare tax of 0.9% that also went into effect in 2013. Employers must withhold the additional Medicare tax from all workers, regardless of marital status, on earnings in excess of $200,000. Thus, the employee Medicare tax rate, normally 1.45%, will rise to 2.35% on earnings higher than $200,000 regardless of the filing status. The employer Medicare tax rate remains 1.45%. There is no

taxable wage limit for Medicare taxes. Remember to always check with your CPA or tax professional or the government website for the most up-to-date tax rates.

- **State income taxes:** The tax percentage varies by state, and several states do not have income taxes. Check with your state for your withholding requirements. As of this writing, states with no state income tax include:
  - Alaska
  - Florida
  - Nevada
  - New Hampshire (investment and interest income only)
  - South Dakota
  - Tennessee (investment and interest income only)
  - Texas
  - Washington
  - Wyoming
- **Federal Unemployment Tax Act:** This tax is paid on the first $7,000 in wages per employee and may be as low as 0.8% depending on the timeliness of submission.
- **State Unemployment Insurance:** This varies depending on the employer's experience rating. Usually, this is paid by the employer, but some states require the employees to contribute to this tax as well.
- **Local taxes:** These vary depending on requirements of the jurisdiction, city, or county.

Tax laws and regulations change frequently and vary widely based on number of staff members, geographic location, exempt status, and regulations. Whether you calculate your payroll in house or contract with an outside accountant or payroll service, it is the employer's responsibility to report and pay taxes based on the federal, state, and local laws. Timeliness and accuracy are critical. Vendors and software will help you calculate accurately, but you have to make sure that deposits are made on time. Inaccurate or late deposits can result in penalties and interest charges. Employers who fail to comply with these requirements may be subject to civil and/or criminal tax penalties.

Other Payroll Liabilities

In the course of creating payroll, the practice incurs a liability covering both the employee and the practice through withholdings for the employee portions of taxes and benefits (resulting in net pay), as well as the accruals for employer responsibilities. These amounts must be paid to the taxing entities, as well as contractors (e.g., health insurance providers).

Withholdings

Withholdings from employee paychecks can include:

- Federal income tax
- Social security
- Medicare tax
- State and local tax withholdings
- Employee portion of the employee benefits
- Retirement plan deferrals and other employee contributions
- Garnishments
- Other

Accruals for Employer Responsibilities

These withholdings cover the employer contributions mirroring the withholdings noted above:

- Social security
- Medicare tax
- Federal and State unemployment taxes
- Employee portion of the employee benefits
- Retirement plan contributions
    - Matching and other mandatory contributions
    - Profit sharing and other discretionary contributions

4.4 Payroll Tax Depositing and Reporting

Taxes must be paid and filed to the appropriate federal and state agencies according to very specific schedules, depending on the tax liability. It is critical for you to determine when and where you need to file in order to avoid penalties.

In general, a practice will need to report the payroll taxes (including income and both employer and employee portions of social security and Medicare) on a quarterly basis on Form 941 (Employer's Quarterly Federal Tax Return). Actual timing depends upon the amount of liability. After you file your first Form 941, you must file a return for each quarter, even if you have no taxes to report, until a final return is filed, as explained in the Instructions to Form 941.

At year end, W-2 forms (Wage and Tax Statements) need to be sent or delivered to each employee, with copies filed with the Social Security Administration and copies held by the employer. In addition, the practice needs to file a W-3 with the W-2, which tells the IRS what was paid to employees and reported on the W-2. For any contract employees, a form 1099 must be filed.

Check with state and local regulations regarding the filing and payment requirements. State unemployment taxes generally must be filed on a quarterly basis. While federal unemployment tax returns are filed annually (form 940), the taxes will probably need to be paid quarterly.

Retirement plan employee and employer contributions are determined as set out in the plan documents, including the Basic Plan Document, the Summary Plan Description, Adoption Agreement, Trust Agreement and IRS Determination Letter, plus any amendments to the plan. The practice's third-party administrator, outside accountant and/or outside payroll company often assists with computations for both the employee deferrals and employer match. This can include profit sharing and other discretionary contributions.

Payment for any employee garnishments will be determined by the court.

In the event of noncompliance with the timely filing of payroll taxes, the assessed penalties can be extreme. Most payroll services indemnify the client if taxes are transmitted late or incorrectly calculated.

Another type of penalty is the *trust fund recovery penalty*. These penalties can be assessed against individuals who are responsible for obtaining and paying the taxes (e.g., accountants, owners, healthcare executives, etc.).

Penalties are nondeductible, so the practice is basically paying taxes on its taxes. A delay in paying taxes should never be considered in financial management.

4.5 Segregation of Duties

As with other financial functions, duties should be separated to avoid the potential for theft/fraud. Some of the more common payroll frauds include timesheet falsification, pay rate falsification, and "ghosts" on payroll.

Hiring decisions, including pay rates, should be made by the supervising individual and approved by their supervisor. The person who approves time and attendance records should not be the same person who prepares the payroll. Any payroll checks should not be distributed by the person who prepares payroll, and the reconciliation of the payroll bank account should not be done by the person who prepares the payroll.

As stated previously, the practice should have policies on who can approve overtime and under what circumstances. Finance should review payroll records for any suspicious withholdings or employees with the same address or social security number.

SAMPLE QUESTIONS

1. **Which document must employees complete in order to accurately withhold taxes?**

   A. Employee application

   B. Form W-4

   C. Signed job description

   D. Non-disclosure form

2. **Which of the following is associated with Form 941?**

   A. Accounts payable

   B. Retirement benefits

   C. Payroll taxes

   D. Health insurance benefit

Answers: 1-B, 2-C

TASK 5: BUDGET CREATION AND MANAGEMENT

5.1 Budget Lifecycle

The healthcare executive, or a key financial representative, usually has overall responsibility for preparing and coordinating the budget. The process is most beneficial when key clinical and administrative personnel, physicians, and other members of the governing body engage in the process and base the budget in the organization's operational and strategic plans.

In smaller practices, the outside accountant may occasionally assist in this process, but in most cases, the role of an outside accountant in the budget process should be purely that of an advisor or facilitator. Key stakeholders within the organization should determine the organization's objectives and manage the related budget process.

As with other key processes, management should communicate the purpose and use of the budget as a management tool that can be used to more effectively delegate responsibility for day to day operations. Often, organizations struggle with budgeting. Issues may include not allowing enough time for the process, overreliance on historical data, or gamesmanship with the budget process that diminishes its effectiveness. These include:

- Budget padding: Submitting costs that the department doesn't truly expect to occur so that performance looks better, i.e., appearance of cost savings. Managers sometimes hedge against adversity by submitting easily obtainable budget amounts, especially when personnel evaluations are largely based on adhering to the budget or when across-the-board cost reductions are anticipated. To guard against padding, healthcare executives may benchmark submitted budget amounts against industry data. Zero-based budgeting (discussed below) may also reduce the potential for padding.
- Use it or lose it: Some in the organization may have the attitude that if a cost center did not spend money allotted in the previous budget, or for a specific period, the option to use that money should be taken away. This is a self-defeating strategy. Delays in using budgeted funds can occur for a variety of justifiable reasons. This leads to budget padding.
- The unachievable budget: Some organizations set a very aggressive budget on the revenue side, cost side, or both. This can set up the organization for financial failure and diminish the credibility of the budgeting process. While padding rarely challenges managers, overly ambitious or even unobtainable budgets fail to motivate and ultimately lead to further disengagement. Because they offer little opportunity to avoid failure, unattainable budgets are more likely to increase anxiety than stimulate motivation or creative thinking.

This is not to say that setting an aggressive but achievable budget isn't a viable strategy. Management needs to be clear about its expectations and the means to achieve them. Research indicates budgets that are challenging but attainable improve performance. Jack Welch, the legendary former chief executive officer of

General Electric, agrees: He claims that challenging budgets energize and motivate managers, unleashing creative, out-of-the-box thinking.[8]

Obtain Data from Department Managers

The healthcare executive (or other designated budget coordinator) reviews the practice's goals and objectives, determines what data are needed, and prepares the working documents necessary for obtaining this information. After communicating the operational and strategic objectives, management should create a standard format for data submission. Many organizations use software specifically designed to support the budgeting process.

As a rule, the healthcare executive should delegate the task of gathering budget amounts to the lowest level appropriate (known as a bottoms-up approach), such as department managers for the cost and expense budgets, as well as the patient accounting manager for revenue amounts. This approach is superior to the "top-down" approach, as it typically creates a more accurate budget and engages those who will be accountable for implementing it.

Due to the sensitive and confidential nature of physician compensation, the healthcare executive or a key financial person normally prepares the provider compensation budget.

Budgeting Methodologies

There is no one best way to prepare a budget, but there are many useful templates you can use, depending on what purpose the budget needs to serve. Except for zero-based budgeting, practices often using prior years' actuals as the place to start.

Fixed vs. Flexible

A fixed budget computes one best estimate for revenues and related expenses. Budget variances are based on differences between actual performance and the estimated set of numbers. A flexible budget assumes that actual results may vary and provides a mechanism for computing budget variances at different volume levels, based on a careful assessment of fixed, step-fixed, and variable costs. The advantage of a flexible budget is its ability to better assess financial performance at different activity levels. The primary disadvantage is that it is more time-consuming.

Traditional vs. Zero-Based

The traditional budget process uses prior and current-year activity levels, revenues, and expenses as a basis for determining prospective values for the coming year. Conversely, zero-based budgeting begins each budget without considering past performance. Essentially, the budget starts at zero and all budget assumptions are reassessed.

The primary disadvantage of zero-based budgeting is that it is more time-consuming than traditional budgeting, With the lack of historic information, you lose the advantage of examining trending data. The major advantage is that, because the zero-based budget process forces a practice to start over, it provides more insights into practice revenues and expenses. Thus, the practice will be more likely to set up its business in such a manner that, by meeting its budget objectives, it will also be successful in achieving its strategic or business plan.

Assemble Budget and Revise as Necessary

After receiving requested data from key clinical and administrative personnel, the healthcare executive and finance leadership assimilates it into a budget form or template. The healthcare executive identifies problem areas and inconsistencies with the numbers as compared to the practice's goals and modifies the budget in coordination with the participants and governing body. Business plan revisions may be necessary if desired physician compensation or other objectives prove incompatible with financial realities.

Board Approval

After assembling a budget that is consistent with the organization's goals and financial realities, the healthcare executive presents it to the governing body for approval. During this approval process, the healthcare executive should be adequately prepared to describe the budget development process that occurred, explain any significant changes, especially market changes that may impact the previous year's or actual results, and make any updates or revisions after board input.

Ongoing Monitoring and Revisions

Throughout the budget period, the practice monitors the actual results versus the budget projections and stays alert for changes in the operating environment that necessitate changes to the budget or operations, developing action plans with specific timelines and tactics needed to address any variances.

To assist practice leadership in monitoring the budget, many accounting systems have report-writing features, such as a comparison of income statement balances against the budget. Most client accounting software packages enable an outside accounting firms to produce these types of statements.

5.2 Types of Budgets

Budgets serve several purposes. Budgets aid in making and coordinating short-range plans and communicating those plans to managers and stakeholders. They provide a mechanism to enable managers to acquire resources in an organized way and can allow them to monitor financial conditions in order to adjust decisions as appropriate. Budgets also establish benchmarks to control ongoing activities and set criteria for evaluating performance.

The major benefit of budgets is that they require managers to plan in an organized and concentrated way. Budgets are short-range targets expressed in financial terms. The process demands that the medical group set aside a specific time each year to plan and that the plans be built on already-established goals and objectives.

Some budgets are simple, while others are more complex. A medical practice should prepare different budgets depending on the mission, approach to management, and organizational culture and structure. Typical budgets that a medical practice may prepare include:

- Provider compensation forecast
- Statistics budget
- Operating budget
- Revenue budget
- Expense budget
- Capital budget
- Cash budget

These budgets form the comprehensive budget that you can present to the practice's governing board to achieve consensus on practice performance and strategy.

Provider Compensation Forecast

The provider compensation forecast is the remainder of revenue after the operating costs and salaries of nonphysician providers and salaried physicians are paid, which is available for distribution to the physician owners and shareholders.

Statistics Budget

The statistics budget, which is also referred to as a service volume forecast, predicts the volume of services a practice can expect to perform. It is the foundation for all other budgets and is crucial to the budgeting process. Often, a practice will assign relative value units (RVUs) to particular services. RVUs help a manager predict a total number of patient visits and can be thought of as a common denominator that relates all services on the same scale. If your practice does not use RVUs, the services might need to be budgeted individually.

Operating Budget

The operating budget includes the revenue and expense budget that predicts the practice's financial performance. In most practices, the operating budget predicts the practice's profit or loss. For planning purposes, apply the formula:

Total Revenue – Total Operating Expenses
– Provider Compensation Forecast = Profit

If the amount calculated is positive, the profit can be pooled into provider compensation. If it is negative, adjustments should be made because physician owners and shareholders will not be paid as expected.

Revenue Budget

The revenue budget is derived from the statistics budget. A healthcare executive should prepare a revenue budget on a monthly basis, which will help predict monthly revenue. The revenue budget includes the practice's ability to collect A/R, depending on the mix of services and the mix of payers.

Expense Budget

The expense budget is also based on the statistics budget. The expense budget focuses on each expense category and includes a labor budget (fixed and variable labor expenses), a supplies budget (non-labor expenses, such as variable costs associated with services), and what the business world refers to as the administrative and general budget (i.e., fixed costs such as interest, depreciation, utilities, rent, cleaning, and housekeeping). The expense budget goes through extensive revisions as projects and staffing levels are approved. Staffing decisions have the greatest effect on the expense budget and should be monitored.

After preparing these budgets, a manager may now calculate expected profit or loss on both an annual and a monthly basis, and decide whether or not the budget satisfies the practice's goals. Once the operating budget is approved, the manager can prepare other key budgets, such as the capital budget and the cash budget.

Capital Budget

A capital budget is necessary if a practice's goals require additional capital expenses. The capital budget summarizes the practice's expectations in acquiring capital assets that have lives greater than one year, such as land, equipment, and other fixed assets. It can be considered a detailed list and acquisition schedule, based on medical necessity or economic benefit to the practice. The return on investment must also be calculated to justify acquisitions.

Cash Budget

The cash budget is a period-to-period estimate of the practice's cash levels. Days in A/R becomes a critical measurement in a managerial cash budget, and this type of aging analysis should be applied to each payer so that you know when you will receive payments that can be used to run the practice. An organization does not want to have too much cash on hand because that would limit opportunities for short-term investment. Too little cash on hand is a problem as well because the practice may need to borrow, which inevitably involves paying interest. Preparing an adequate cash budget involves looking at the expense budget, the revenue budget, the practice's balance sheet from the previous year, and an aging analysis.

SAMPLE QUESTIONS

1. **What is the purpose of a budget?**
   A. To manage cash flow
   B. To provide a quantitative expression of a plan for a defined period of time
   C. To plan for long-term capital purchases over multiple accounting periods
   D. To provide a baseline for comparison of performance over time

2. **Which is the foundation for all other budgets?**
   A. Expense budget
   B. Statistics budget
   C. Operations budget
   D. Revenue budget

3. **Budgets can be most useful for strategic and operational planning because they enable the healthcare executive to:**
   A. Explain variances after they have occurred
   B. Identify unfavorable trends to minimize their future impact
   C. Learn best practices about how practice finances work
   D. Show off their financial acumen to the board of directors

Answers: 1-B, 2-B, 3-B

TASK 6: FINANCIAL REPORTING

KEY TERMS

Balance sheet: Lists the medical group's assets balanced by the liability claims of creditors and the residual owners' equity.

Capital financing: Institutional funding for facilities and for equipment, which becomes a part of the assets of the institution.

Capital gain: The amount by which an asset's selling price exceeds its initial purchase price. A realized capital gain is an investment that has been sold at a profit. An unrealized capital gain is an investment that hasn't been sold yet but would result in a profit if sold.

Current assets: Cash and other assets that can be converted into cash within one year.

Current liabilities: Obligations arising from past transactions that must be paid by using current assets or by creating other current liabilities.

Depreciation: Gradual conversion of the cost of a tangible capital asset or fixed asset into an operational expense over the asset's estimated useful life.

Distributions: The payment of a dividend or capital gain.

Equity: Depending on the legal structure of an organization, owner's equity may include contributed capital, undistributed earnings, different classes of stock, donated capital, or retained earnings. In general, stockholder's equity (or the related capital accounts for an unincorporated entity) represents the difference between assets and liabilities on the balance sheet.

Income statement: Conveys information about the accomplishments of the practice, measured in revenue dollars, matched with related efforts, and measured by goods and services consumed, or expenses. By comparing income statements for several consecutive periods, significant trends in statement components can be identified, and projections about the practice's future earning power can be made.

Intangibles and other assets: Organization costs, goodwill, and relocation costs.

Investments: Restricted cash, long-term receivables, investments in securities, investments in affiliates, and property held for future use.

Long-term liabilities: Obligations that will not mature and will not require the use of current assets within one year of the balance sheet date. The major types are long-term notes payable, mortgages, capital lease obligations, and deferred income taxes.

continued on next page

Losses: The opposite of a capital gain. The amount by which an asset's current value is less than its purchase value.

Net income: The residual amount after all expenses — operating and nonoperating — have been deducted from net revenue and nonoperating revenue.

Variance analysis: Profit variance analysis highlights the financial factors responsible for the discrepancy between estimated and actual profits and leads to focused investigation.

6.1 Accounting Systems and Software

An accounting system provides the basic structure for accumulating the practice's financial information. The amounts contained in financial statements and tax returns come from the accounting system. Historical information from the accounting system may be used to determine the amounts used in prospective statements, such as budgets and forecasts. Even if a practice uses zero-based budgeting and derives its budget from scratch, it still compares this budget against actual data from the accounting system.

The accounting system does not just provide information for financial reporting, it also supplies much of the information used for decision-making. For example, determining the break-even point or computing the cost of sending out a bill involves using data from the accounting system. The information used to compute physician bonuses or track expense accounts also comes from the accounting system.

An accounting system begins with a chart of accounts, which categorizes the various transactions that are recorded through payroll, A/P, the revenue cycle, and other sources. The transactions are then posted to the general ledger, which lists the activity for each account number in the chart of accounts and maintains the balance of cumulative activity for each account. The amounts from the general ledger provide the basis for the financial statements, tax returns, and many financial analyses.

It is critical for the healthcare executive to have strong a financial acumen and to closely monitor both the funds generated by the practice and those being paid by the practice. It is crucial to have the right accounting software in place, integrated with the medical practice billing software, to create a seamless system of generating claims, recording revenue, paying invoices, tracking expenses, and reconciling every transaction. A high-functioning system allows the healthcare executive to generate reports that measure the practice's financial health using a variety of metrics.

The key questions facing practice leadership when choosing the right accounting software are:

- How much to pay for accounting software? This depends, in large part, on the features the practice needs.
- How many users will need access to the system and what platforms are necessary to maximize their productivity? Accounting systems can be managed in a traditional desktop environment, on a cloud-based environment or via a mobile app.
- What does the system need to do? What are the types and volumes of transactions required and what types of reports will the practice need?

6.2 Generally Accepted Accounting Principles (GAAP)

Before delving into the chart of accounts, it is important to understand the basic financial statements that your practice needs to create on a regular basis. These include the:

- Balance sheet
- Income statement
- Statement of changes in equity
- Statement of cash flows

These financial statements may be prepared using the accrual basis of accounting in accordance with generally accepted accounting principles (GAAP) or some other comprehensive basis of accounting (OCBOA), such as the cash or tax basis.

6.3 Chart of Accounts

A standard chart of accounts is a numbered list of accounts that comprise a practice's general ledger. It serves as a filing system for classifying all transactions during a specific accounting period, broken down into categories. The chart of accounts forms the foundation for the practice's entire financial reporting system.

A physician practice uses its chart of accounts to organize its finances, which gives the physicians or other parties a clearer insight into its financial health. Dividing the information into revenue, expenditures, assets, and liabilities ensures that the financial statements are in compliance with generally accepted accounting principles.[9] In addition, a well-conceived chart of accounts helps the healthcare executive track every type of transaction, be able to quickly calculate variances by account, and respond accordingly.

For a typical physician practice, a chart of accounts would include these categories, with additional subcategories within each one:

- Assets
- Liabilities
- Owner's equity
- Revenues
- Cost of goods sold
- Operating expenses

6.4 Cash and Accrual Accounting and Modified Accrual Accounting

Medical practices generally use either the cash or the accrual method of accounting. The accrual method of accounting is consistent with GAAP. The basic and most important difference between the cash and accrual methods is the point at which each recognizes revenues and expenses. Accrual-basis organizations recognize revenues when they are earned and expenses when they are incurred. Cash-basis organizations recognize revenue when the cash is actually or constructively received and expenses when they are actually or constructively paid.

For a medical practice, this means that an accrual-basis practice includes medical revenue on its income statement and the net value of any related A/R on its balance sheet at the time the physician sees the patient. A cash-basis practice includes the revenue from the visit in its income statement when it receives payment for the services. It never shows the related A/R on its balance sheet.

6.5 Elements of Financial Statements

Balance Sheets

The balance sheet tells what the practice owns (its assets), what it owes (its liabilities), and its net worth of equity (its net claim on assets after subtracting liabilities). True to its name, the balance sheet must balance. The balance sheet equation is:

Assets = Liabilities + Equity

A balance sheet lists the assets and liabilities in the order of their liquidity (how quickly they convert to cash). The most liquid assets and liabilities are called current assets and liabilities because they are expected to convert to cash in less than one year. Examples of current assets include cash and accounts receivable (A/R). Examples of current liabilities include A/P, payroll withholdings and accruals, and current maturities of long-term debt. Any long-term investments would appear in a separate section between current assets and property and equipment.

Balance Sheet: Assets

Assets are resources owned by the organization, such as A/R, equipment, and property. Assets may be tangible, such as land, buildings, and equipment, or intangible, such as goodwill, patents owned by the organization, and licenses. The chart of accounts lists assets in descending order of liquidity. Cash and other assets that are easily converted to cash are listed first, fixed assets such as property and equipment are listed next, and intangible assets are listed last.

A practice's long-term assets usually consist of medical equipment and other property, such as computers, office furniture, and leasehold improvements. The balance sheet shows these items in a separate section, along with their cumulative depreciation and net book value.

Other long-term assets are those with an expected life greater than one year, other than investments, property, and equipment. These are included in the last group in the assets section. Examples include deposits and intangible assets, such as goodwill.

Balance Sheet: Liabilities

Liabilities are debts or obligations owed by the practice to creditors, such as loans and A/P. These obligations come from the purchase of goods or services on credit, or by obtaining a loan from a financial institution to finance the purchase of equipment or buildings. Current liabilities, the obligations that are due to be paid within one year, are generally listed first in the chart of accounts, with A/P, bank overdrafts payable, and payroll obligations (tax, insurance, retirement plan withholdings, and accrued payroll amounts) listed before other payables such as rent or insurance. Long-term liabilities such as construction loans, long-term notes, and capital leases follow current liabilities.

Long-term liabilities appear in a separate section, following the current liabilities. These include debts that the practice will pay in one year or more, such as long-term debt and net of current maturities. The equity section represents the owners' claim on net assets.

These amounts are the result of capital contributed by the owners, as well as the undistributed profits of the practice. The accounts in this section will vary depending on the type of entity. For example, corporate entities will show all classes of stock separately at par value, beginning with common stock and followed by any contributed capital in excess of par and by retained earnings. Limited liability entities, partnerships, and sole proprietorships generally combine these amounts as members' capital, partners' capital, or proprietor's capital. Although one amount usually appears in these entities' balance sheets for capital, practices should keep detailed subaccounts for each owner.

Balance Sheet: Equity Accounts

Equity accounts (sometimes called fund balance in nonprofit organizations) reflect the net financial worth of the organization and represent the residual value of an entity's assets after deducting its liabilities. In a for-profit business, the equity will be the ownership interest. In a not-for-profit, it will represent the retained net asset value of the organization.

The retained earnings or owners' capital accounts should include the current-year net income, not just the undistributed amounts from prior years. This is true not only for the year-end financial statements, but also for interim statements. The related computation (adding current net income from the income statement to the equity account) is shown in the statement of changes in equity and posted to the balance sheet. This is the secret to balancing the balance sheet.

Income Statement: Revenue and Expenses

The accounts used to create the income statement follow the statement of financial position accounts. The accounts used to describe operating revenue precede the expense accounts, and the final accounts reflect non-operating revenue, non-operating expenses, and income taxes.

Revenues are inflows of cash and other items of value received by the practice. Different revenue accounts categorize income to the practice by source, whether it is from fee-for-service activity, the sale of medical material, capitation payment, or some other source.

Expenses reflect the resources consumed in the process of generating revenue for the practice. Operating expenses include support staff salaries and benefits, and the cost of temporary labor; general and administrative expenses; clinical and ancillary services expenses; physician and non-physician provider expenses; and nonmedical revenue and expenses.

Whereas the balance sheet shows the practice's assets, liabilities, and equity at a point in time, the income statement shows the entity's revenue, expenses, and net income over a period of time. The basic equation for the income statement is:

Revenues – Expenses = Net Income or (Loss)

The standard accounting period is one year. Any audit or review by an outside accounting firm would generally be performed on the annual financial statements. Ordinarily, a practice will also prepare interim financial statements on a monthly basis showing current month- and year-to-date amounts on the income statement.

Operating revenues, such as fee-for-service income, capitation income, and other medical revenue, such as medical director fees, appear first on the income statement. GAAP requires that any significant amount of capitation revenue be shown separately from fee-for-service income.

The operating expenses appear next. These expenses relate directly to the production of operating revenues. Both GAAP and OCBOA allow an entity to organize, classify, and sub-classify these expenses in a useful or customary manner. One method that works well for most medical practices is to divide these expenses into staff salaries and fringe benefits, services and general expenses, purchased services, and provider-related expenses.

The income statement also includes income and expenses from sources other than operations: These include investment incomes, gains or losses on the sale of used medical equipment, and interest expense. Finally, after deducting income taxes, the income statement shows the practice's net income.

Statement of Changes in Equity

The statement of changes in equity shows the activity in the capital accounts during the period and includes changes in both contributed capital and accumulated earnings accounts. Practices whose changes consist only of net earnings and distributions to owners often combine this statement with the income statement.

Groups with more complex equity transactions, such as shareholder buy-ins or buyouts, generally report these transactions in a separate statement.

Statement of Cash Flow

The statement of cash flow explains the practice's sources and uses of cash during the year. The three categories are cash provided or used by:

1. Operating activities (the practice's normal business activities)
2. Investing activities (sales and purchases of investments, including equipment and other fixed assets)
3. Financing activities (transactions involving the practice's debt and equity)

All of the entity's cash transactions fit into one of these three categories. The statement can present the section on operating activities using either the direct or indirect method.

Financial Statement Preparation

The amounts on a practice's balance sheet and its income statement come directly from its general ledger. Often, the balances of similar accounts are combined to create one line item on the financial statements. For example, a practice may have several cash accounts, but only one amount for cash on its balance sheet. To prepare the statement of cash flows, accounting personnel must go beyond the general ledger and analyze cash flow and/or other account activity. Preparing the statement of changes in equity may also involve additional analysis.

Presenting Financial Results to Stakeholders

Although the healthcare executive frequently performs much of the practice's financial analysis, physicians and other stakeholders often have the ultimate responsibility for practice activities and major financial decisions. For example, the governing body anticipates cash flow and assesses management's performance. It makes crucial decisions on whether to add another physician, buy a building, offer ancillary services, and many other issues.

To fulfill these responsibilities, decision-makers need timely and relevant information on the practice's financial performance. On some occasions, they may need special analyses such as an ROI or cost-benefit. The healthcare executive must ensure that these stakeholders not only receive this information, but that they understand it well enough to make informed decisions. This task can be especially challenging when some decision-makers have limited financial knowledge. At the same time, however, the healthcare executive must present enough financial detail to those stakeholders who are financially astute.

6.6 Projections and Proforma Financial Statements

The executive should provide agreed-upon financial reports to physicians and other stakeholders on a regular basis. These normally include financial statements, budget comparisons, billing information, and clinical productivity metrics. Depending on the nature of the practice, stakeholders may want other reports, such as incoming/outgoing referrals, cancellations and no-shows, or appointment availability. Providing a dashboard of summary financial data gives a high-level summary of practice performance.

Some of the most important reporting projects are those special reports that the healthcare executive prepares on an as-needed basis to facilitate a particular decision, such as whether to invest in an electronic health record system or whether to change the way the group's employee health insurance is handled.

Forecast Trend and Variance Reporting

Forecasting is a planning tool that helps cope with the uncertainty of the future, relying mainly on data from the past and present and analysis of trends. Forecasting starts with certain assumptions based on experience, knowledge, and judgment. These estimates are projected into the coming months or years. A forecast should not be confused with a budget.

Trend analysis is a method of analysis involving comparison of the same item (such as monthly revenue figures) over a significantly long period to detect the general pattern of a relationships between associated factors or variables, and to project the future direction of this pattern.

A variance is the difference between a budgeted, planned, or standard cost and the actual amount incurred or sold. Variances can be computed for both costs and revenues. The concept of variance is intrinsically connected with planned and actual results and the effects of the difference between those two on the performance of the entity or company.

Manage Short-Term Investments

Assets that are closely related to cash are the short-term cash investments that medical groups enter into for short periods of time.

When the cash position is being built up to meet a large, planned expenditure later in the year, the cash in excess of normal needs should be invested for a return. These temporary excesses in the cash account can be transferred to the group's savings account or into other short-term investments and then returned to cash when needed later. The most frequently mentioned types of investments that groups select are savings accounts, certificates of deposit, U.S. Treasury bills and notes, money market mutual funds, and commercial paper.

The primary characteristics of these investment options are their short-term maturity dates (one year or less) and the ability for the investors to convert back into cash with a minimum of effort and with less risk of losing their original investment amount. Financial managers must be careful in selecting short-term investments, as safety of principal is the paramount concern.

To incorporate any short-term investments into the cash management process, it is important that these investments are monitored, and the amounts of their current values are developed when these investment balances are needed for planning purposes. Each investment should be listed on a schedule that includes the following information:

- Current market value
- Purchase and maturity date (if applicable)
- Income to date
- Yield percentage

Also, the total investment balances for the current and previous months should be made available. This information can be used in preparing short-term cash forecasts if investments are to be liquidated within the month. If they are not, their proceeds should be included in the cash budget for the month in which they are liquidated.

Conduct and Communicate Utilization Analyses

Utilization review describes the set of techniques used by healthcare professionals, insurance companies, and the government to evaluate the necessity, appropriateness, and efficiency of care. At its core, the utilization review process seeks to eliminate the duplication of medical services and inappropriate utilization. In most contracts, the physician and/or medical group is required to participate in a utilization review program and quality assurance activities, and to abide by the terms, conditions, and operations of such programs. Even participation is a necessity.

The medical group must not blindly agree to the utilization review measures and quality assurance activities suggested by the managed care entity. In many instances, the managed care agreement will require participation but not provide details on how such programs will be implemented. There should be some agreement and detailed illustrations of the procedures the medical group will be obligated to follow, and of the physicians' responsibilities to comply with the intentions of the program. Much of this information is embedded in the physician manual that is considered part of the contract.

It is important that the group's physicians be involved in the approval process of any utilization review activities outlined in the contract, and that the physician manual and any other supporting documentation referred to in the contract also be reviewed in advance of contract execution. Furthermore, medical groups should seek a contract clause that enables the group to observe the utilization review programs and quality assurance activities currently undertaken by other contracted physicians to ensure that they are consistent with the standards of care rendered by the group.

Forecast Capital Needs

Most medical groups need, or will need, capital. How much capital and for what purposes is often determined by how aggressive the group is or plans to become. Those groups with an aggressive long-term orientation are almost certain to need substantial amounts of capital, and those that are aggressive but with a shorter-term perspective will also benefit from outside financing. Retained earnings, debt financing, and leasing are often insufficient for the more aggressive types of medical groups.

There are 10 common needs for capital:

1. Growing and optimizing the existing practice
2. Adding primary care physicians and sites
3. Investing in new profit centers
4. Adding next-generation facilities and equipment
5. Adding next-generation information systems
6. Developing single-specialty networks
7. Accepting and managing medical risk
8. Providing an exit strategy for older physicians
9. Covering cash flow shortages
10. Insulating against risk

Conduct Financial Analysis

Healthcare executives must obtain meaningful data quickly. Financial analysis can take the form of profitability measures; profitability ratios; current and prior period comparison; comparisons by department, location, and division; and productivity analysis. Which reports do healthcare executives really need? Key indicator reports compare results and highlight variances. The following subsections highlight a few examples, although it's important to remember that this is not an exhaustive list.

Actual Weekly Charges Per Provider and Business Unit

An executive may not know about problems in clinic operations until after end-of-month reports. These reports are normally ready five to 10 working days after the end of the month — when it is too late to make significant changes to the functions of the current month.

Unless the healthcare executive receives key indicator reports promptly, the operation of the practice can deteriorate. With a daily report that accumulates month-to-date charges and collections per provider, business unit, and total practice, the healthcare executive can act promptly.

Monthly budgeted charges and collections are derived from the annual budget and can be compared to actual numbers. A report that shows daily and month-to-date charges allows an executive to pinpoint problems with charge production or charge entry.

Payer Mix for the Practice, Each Provider, or Business Unit

At the end of each month, most billing systems generate reports for charges, collections, and A/R. The system should issue a report giving the charges per provider or business unit for major categories such as Medicare, Medicaid, commercial insurance, managed care, self-pay, and others. Determine the percentage of each category for the total practice and for each provider and produce trends for the data over 12 months.

Calculate a payer mix report for collections in the same manner. This permits a quick look at the payer sources constituting the practice's portfolio. Even in a single-specialty practice with more than one provider and/or location, payer mix reports may fluctuate considerably. Prepare a report for each business unit.

Review fluctuations each month. Pay close attention to this report, especially after January, when companies typically implement new health plans for the calendar year. Develop professional relationships with the benefit directors of your area's major employers to learn — before the end of the previous calendar year — their chosen health plans. The group might want to lobby major employers for the best health plan in the area.

Payer mix reports provide a baseline for plan marketing efforts. They also allow the practice to keep a well-balanced portfolio of payer categories.

Collections and Collection Rate for Each Provider and Business Unit

Any billing system will provide actual collections per day, month-to-date, and year-to-date. These numbers should allow for a variance analysis against the budgeted figures. Budgeting a gross collection rate per provider and for the entire practice — calculated by dividing gross collections by gross charges — permits a quick analysis of collection efforts.

Anemic collections may reflect inadequate charges and collection efforts, poorly managed contracts, or inefficient operations. This report, together with charge analysis, payer mix review, and an analysis of A/R will give a quick indication of potential problems.

Trended Value of Accounts Receivable for the Medical Practice

When reviewing the net value of A/R, look at the trends from month to month by major payer category, such as commercial, Medicare, Medicaid, managed care, self-pay, and others. This report will determine:

- A/R turnover
- Occurrence of bad debt after a set limit, such as 180 days
- How credit balances affect the net A/R
- Days that receivables are outstanding
- Percentage distribution of receivables within a certain set of parameters, such as 80% less than 90 days and 20% more than 90 days

You can obtain net receivables by determining a percentage adjudication rate for a practice for a set of charges over a 12- to 18-month period.

Monthly Costs by Provider and Business Unit

A perennial problem in the healthcare industry has been its inability to quickly ascertain the cost of doing business. Knowing costs is the highest priority before your group negotiates with a managed care company. Set up your systems to capture data and produce reports promptly.

Assign one account per provider or business unit to log all associated costs. This is initially time-consuming but pays off in the long run. Some physicians tend to spend big. It takes discipline and systematic strategies to keep the practice within bounds. A budget that can account for each provider's contributions to expenses will allow the practice to spot problems and/or opportunities. Each clinic should have its own cost center to capture personnel and operational expenses.

Budgets that can track cost centers allow for accurate and speedy input processes. A cost center is assigned to each expense even before the expense is incurred. If the practice accounting system allows it, make every effort to treat all expenses on an accrual basis. Accrued payroll and fixed monthly costs allow for fast expenditure projections through year-end. Knowing costs per provider and/or business unit will let you determine cost per RVUs and other important financial ratios.

Actual vs. Budgeted Net Balance Per Provider and Business Unit

A responsible executive sets up net balances for each provider or business unit. The net balance incorporates revenues and expenses. This report challenges each provider to analyze the net balance (actual amount versus budgeted amount), regardless of the method used for distributing the overhead amounts.

Providers need to understand cost behavior, since their production and decision-making impact these costs. For example, a provider who brings in the highest collections will likely also use the most resources, due to increased variable costs, such as medical supplies. Each business unit accounts for its own revenues and direct expenditures. Direct expenditures include physician salaries and benefits; support staff directly assigned to physicians; malpractice costs; and other physician expenses, such as travel, membership dues, cellular phones, conference registrations, and entertainment.

Several models allocate overhead based on charges, collections, expenses, RVUs, or activity-based costing methods. Once a group decides to account for each business unit by tracking its direct revenues and expenses, and once it allocates its overhead expenditures, each unit has a budgeted net balance.

Conduct Financial Benchmarking

Medical practices may benchmark their performance against that of similar practices, which includes looking at revenue, expenses, adjusted collection rate, collection rate by payer, payer mix, reimbursement, productivity, A/R, and profitability. Limitations in benchmarking against industry data may occur if a practice has different characteristics than your practice. Another way to benchmark is to compare current year results for the similar time period. You will need to take into consideration several variables such as changes in physicians, procedure types, volume, and/or payer mix.

Key performance indicators denote highlights of performance for significant aspects of the practice. Some are financial and others are nonfinancial. Key indicators include measures such as number of full-time equivalents per physician, total operating costs per physician, gross collection ratio, total net revenue per physician, and many others.

Communicate Financial Information to Stakeholders

The purpose of both financial and operational reporting is to convey accurate information effectively and guide action. The hallmarks of effective reporting include brevity, clarity, timeliness, and accuracy. The modes of communication can include graphs, narratives, presentations, dashboards, scorecards, and executive summaries.

When you're presenting practice data to providers, keep the visual presentation as simple as possible and try to focus on the most important data points. Use color selectively to emphasize a point.

Examples of a dashboard include:

- Operational dashboards for information needed daily
- Tactical dashboards to focus on trends
- Strategic dashboards to display big-picture data and goals

A useful revenue cycle approach requires developing a robust dashboard report with key billing metrics. The report should include daily and weekly charges, gross collections, net collection rates, and denial percentages. The report can also include data on physician quality reporting measures required for Medicare incentive payments under the Physician Quality Reporting System. It should break down data by payer and provider, and the dashboard should include monthly roll-ups along with month-to-month and year-to-year comparisons.

A well-constructed dashboard report allows you to quickly evaluate performance throughout your revenue cycle and identify problems. For example, the dashboard's denial metrics might show that a payer has rejected claims with a certain physical status modifier for the last three months. Detecting this problem through your dashboard gives you the opportunity to investigate the cause of the problem, prevent it from recurring, and possibly recoup rejected payments.

SAMPLE QUESTIONS

1. **What is the primary tool used to evaluate financial performance within a medical practice?**

   A. Capital budget

   B. Supplies budget

   C. Operating budget

   D. Personal budget

2. **What should be used to calculate contribution margin?**

   A. Gross charges only

   B. Gross charges and variable costs

   C. Fixed costs only

   D. Fixed costs and operating income

3. **Examples of fixed costs within a medical practice include:**

   A. Physician bonuses

   B. Medication/drug costs

   C. Rent/lease fees

   D. Medical supply expense

4. **It is important to have a segregation of duties, particularly relating to the practice's financial management, to ensure the following:**

   A. One staff member doesn't get bored with the same routine every day

   B. In case someone is out for an extended period of time, it's a good opportunity for many staff members to learn the processes

   C. Avoidance of the potential for fraud and abuse by having internal controls in place

   D. The finance department can rely on many team members to do their work

Answers: 1-C, 2-B, 3-C, 4-C

TASK 7: AUDIT MANAGEMENT

7.1 Types of Audits

There are several types of audits:

- An independent examination of an organization's financial statements is called a **financial audit**. Financial audits are usually performed by independent accountants, generally CPAs.
- An **operational audit** is performed to determine the extent to which some aspect of an organization's operating activity is functioning effectively and efficiently.
- A **compliance audit** determines the extent to which an organization and its employees are performing their duties in a manner consistent with organizational policies or in compliance with federal laws, regulations, contracts, and grants.
- A **billing audit** ensures that the amounts of net revenue (fee-for-service revenue, capitation revenue, pay for performance, and any other revenues) in the financial statements present a reasonably accurate representation of the amounts the practice will ultimately collect.
- A **forensic audit** is an examination and evaluation of an organization's financial records to derive evidence that can be used in a court of law or legal proceeding. Forensic auditing is a specialization within the field of accounting, and most large accounting firms have a forensic auditing department.

7.2 Financial Statement Reports

Audit examinations are carried out following a prescribed set of standards that measure the quality of the auditor's performance as well as the objectives to be attained by using certain procedures. These auditing standards rarely change, and if they do, it's only by the official decree of the Auditing Standards Board, a professional body of CPAs who constantly monitor the effectiveness of existing standards and developments. Generally accepted auditing standards (GAAS) are important for several reasons:

- To define the broad objectives of every independent audit
- To provide a gauge for judging an auditor's performance
- To set recognized standards of the profession throughout the business and legal world

There are 10 GAAS, which are divided into three broad categories:

(1) General standards
(2) Standards of fieldwork
(3) Standards of reporting

These standards, as developed by the Auditing Standards Board and approved by the members of the American Institute of Certified Public Accountants

(AICPA, the professional organization of CPAs), are listed in Exhibit 2.3. Financial managers should be aware of these standards when they assess their practice's internal and external auditing services.

Auditors' reports are addressed to the governing body of the organization requesting the audit. An introductory paragraph identifies the responsibilities of both the client (e.g., XYZ Company) and the auditor regarding the financial statements. The second paragraph contains the auditor's description of the scope of the examination and is called the *scope paragraph*. In the third paragraph, the auditor renders an opinion about the fairness of the presentation of the financial statements in what is usually referred to as the *opinion paragraph*. The report is signed by a partner of the CPA firm involved. The date printed on the report is the actual date the audit fieldwork was completed. This indicates the point at which the auditor was in a position to render an opinion.

An unqualified audit opinion, illustrated in Exhibit 2.4, means that the auditor believes that the financial statements are presented fairly, that they conform with GAAP, that they are applied consistently each year, and that the statements include all necessary disclosures. It means that the statements fairly present the financial position, results of operations, and cash flows.

Besides the unqualified opinion, auditors can render three other types of opinions:

1. A qualified opinion in which the auditor expresses certain reservations in the report regarding the scope of the audit and/or the financial statements. When the auditor's reservations are more serious, one of the two following types of opinions are rendered.
2. A *disclaimer of opinion* in which auditors state that they cannot give an opinion because of scope limitations (e.g., the auditor has been precluded from completing certain significant audit procedures) or some other reason (e.g., the auditor is not independent).
3. An *adverse opinion* in which the auditors state that the financial statements do not fairly present the financial position of the company, the results of its operations, and the cash flows. In this case, it is claimed that the client is making a serious departure from GAAP.

EXHIBIT 2.3

Generally Accepted Auditing Standards[10]

General Standards

1. The auditor must have adequate technical training and proficiency to perform the audit.
2. The auditor must maintain independence in mental attitude in all matters relating to the audit.
3. The auditor must exercise due professional care in the performance of the audit and the preparation of the auditor's report.

Standards of Fieldwork

4. The auditor must adequately plan the work and must properly supervise any assistants.
5. The auditor must obtain a sufficient understanding of the entity and its environment, including its internal control, to assess the risk of material misstatement of the financial statements whether due to error or fraud, and to design the nature, timing, and extent of further audit procedures.
6. The auditor must obtain sufficient appropriate audit evidence by performing audit procedures to afford a reasonable basis for an opinion regarding the financial statements under audit.

Standards of Reporting

7. The auditor must state in the auditor's report whether the financial statements are presented in accordance with generally accepted accounting principles.
8. The auditor must identify in the auditor's report those circumstances in which such principles have not been consistently observed in the current period in relation to the preceding period.
9. If the auditor determines that informative disclosures in the financial statements are not reasonably adequate, the auditor must so state in the auditor's report.
10. The auditor's report must either express an opinion regarding the financial statements, taken as a whole, or state that an opinion cannot be expressed. When the auditor cannot express an overall opinion, the auditor should state the reasons in the auditor's report. In all cases where an auditor's name is associated with financial statements, the auditor should clearly indicate the character of the auditor's work, if any, and the degree of responsibility the auditor is taking, in the auditor's report.

EXHIBIT 2.4

Standard Auditor's Report: Example of an Unqualified Audit Opinion[11]

"We have audited the accompanying balance sheet of XYZ Company as of December 31, 2XXX, and the related statements of income, retained earnings, and cash flows for the year then ended. These financial statements are the responsibility of the company's management. Our responsibility is to express an opinion on these financial statements based on our audit.

"We conducted our audit based on generally accepted auditing standards. Those standards require that we plan and perform the audit to obtain reasonable assurance about whether the financial statements are free of material misstatement. An audit includes examining, on a test basis, evidence supporting the amounts and disclosures in the financial statements. An audit also includes assessing the accounting principles used and significant estimates made by management as well as evaluating the overall financial statement presentation. We believe that our audit provides a reasonable basis for our opinion.

"In our opinion, the financial statements above present fairly, in all material respects, the financial position of XYZ Company as of December 31, 2XXX, and the results of its operations and its cash flow for the year ended in conformity with generally accepted accounting principles."

SAMPLE QUESTIONS

1. **Which type of audit deals specifically with legal concerns?**
   A. Financial
   B. Operational
   C. Forensic
   D. Billing

2. **What does an unqualified opinion on audited financial statements indicate?**
   A. That the auditors found no errors in the financial statements
   B. That the auditors discovered no fraud in conducting the audit
   C. That the auditors found the financial statements to be free of material misstatement
   D. That the auditors were unable to obtain enough information to complete the audit

Answers: 1-C, 2-C

TASK 8: CORPORATE TAX REPORTING

Medical practices find themselves subject to multiple, federal, state, and local taxes. The healthcare executive must assure that taxes are paid accurately and on time. While the approach to federal taxes does not vary by location, state and local taxes will. Make sure to know the specific requirements for your state and locality. This section should serve as a guide but cannot substitute for expert counsel. A tax accountant or attorney will have the expertise you may require from time to time.

Types of Corporate Taxes

The types of tax liability for your practice will vary based not only on your location but the type of organization/entity. For example, if organized as a partnership, the individual partners/owners will be liable for income taxes, unlike a corporation, which pays taxes directly before distributing profits. And some practices may be organized as a not-for-profit entity and as a result, while generally not required to pay federal income taxes, will still have a sales/use tax liability, for example. In fact, sometimes not-for-profits may owe federal taxes for Unrelated Business Income (UBI) which encompasses income from any activity substantially unrelated to furthering the not-for-profit's purposes.

Figure 2.1[12] describes the types of legal structures and their tax implications. As a reminder, your tax accountant or tax attorney should be consulted as to the best solution in your position.

Figure 2.1

Issue	**C Corporation**	**S Corporation**
Number of owners	One or more	One to 100
Limited liability (except malpractice)	Yes	Yes
Tax on entity income paid by	Entity	Generally, owners (exception for built-in gains and excessive passive income)
Double taxation	Yes	Not usually, with exception for built-in gains and excessive passive income)
Entity tax reporting form	Form 1120	Form 1120S (includes Form 1120S K-1 for each owner)
Physician-owner tax reporting	N/A	Include share of income and deductions from their 1120S K-1 in Schedule E of Form 1040
Debt basis for pass-through losses and deductions	N/A	Must be loan directly from shareholder to the S corporation
Unreasonable compensation issue	Yes	No, except for payroll taxes when compensation deemed too low
Exclusion of certain fringe benefits (e.g., health, disability, long-term care, $50,000 group term life insurance) from owner income	Yes	No for > 2% owners who may be able to deduct some of all health and long-term care insurance separately on individual income tax returns

Overview of Federal Taxes

The United States Federal Government requires medical groups to pay income taxes on revenues less expenses. Figure 2.1 provides an overview of federal tax implications.

Estimated Taxes

C corporations must generally make estimated tax payments on a quarterly basis if their tax liability is greater than $500, or pay penalties. Although the owners will usually pay the taxes for S corporation income on their individual tax returns, an S corporation may need to make estimated tax payments for certain types of tax. Similarly, tax-exempt corporations may encounter situations in which they are required to make estimated tax payments. These payments should be made on a pro rata basis throughout the year, although exceptions may apply for seasonal or annualized income adjustments. Exceptions may also be available for corporations that make estimated payments based on their prior year income taxes; however, the entity must have incurred a prior year tax liability to use this exception.

Limited Liability Entity	Partnership	Sole Proprietorship
LLC – One or more; LLP – two or more	Two or more	One
Yes	No	No
Consistent with form of tax entity selected	Owners	Owners
Consistent with form of tax entity selected	No	No
Consistent with form of tax entity selected	Form 1065 (includes Form 1065 K-1 for each owner)	Reports practice income and expenses on Schedule C of their Form 1040
Consistent with form of tax entity selected	Include share of income and deductions from their 1065 K-1 in Schedule E of Form 1040	Reports practice income and expenses on Schedule C of Form 1040
Consistent with form of tax entity selected	Yes	Yes
Consistent with form of tax entity selected	No	No
Consistent with form of tax entity selected	No, but may be able to deduct some or all health and long-term care insurance on individual tax returns	No, but may be able to deduct some or all health and long-term care insurance on individual tax returns

If a practice owes state income taxes, estimated taxes will most likely apply here as well. The practice's outside accountant will usually prepare the estimated tax forms for the practice. The individuals in the practice with responsibility for making these deposits should mark their calendars to ensure these are paid on time.

Physician owners of partnerships, sole proprietorships, and limited liability entities taxed as partnerships will generally need to make estimated tax payments for their individual income tax liability, which includes their liability for taxes on entity income. Physician owners of S corporations and LLCs taxed as S corporations will need to make estimated tax payments if the income tax withheld on their paychecks is not enough to cover the required estimated taxes.

Overview of State and Local Taxes

State Income Taxes

Given the significant variability among the states, please refer to the website for your state and/or consult your tax accountant or attorney for more complete information.

Adjustments from Federal to State Taxable Income

Often the state tax return will begin by using the reported Federal Taxable Income and then adjust that income through a series of adjustments from Federal Taxable Income to State Taxable Income. These adjustments vary depending upon the state. Some examples include:

- Differences in depreciation: For example, the state may not allow some of the accelerated depreciation methods allowed on the federal income tax return
- Subtracting interest from U.S. securities, such as Treasury bonds, which is not taxable by the states
- Differences in recognition of net operating losses and related carryovers
- Adding back interest earned on bonds issued by other states

States usually require that a copy of the federal tax return be attached to and submitted with the state income tax return.

Apportionment of Income for Taxpayers Operating in Multiple States

Organizations that operate in multiple states need to complete schedules apportioning their income on the various state returns. Each state return will have its own apportionment schedule. The apportionment is usually based on percentage of sales, payroll, and property in that state as compared to total sales, payroll, and property everywhere. Pass-through entities would generally also need to make this computation; the individual owners then report their share of state income on the individual tax returns they file in the various states.

Rules as to when a taxpayer would have a "nexus" in a state and be required to file a tax return in that state vary from state to state. The practice should consult with a tax attorney and/or tax accountant if they believe they may be required to file a return in another state.

State Income Tax Returns for Pass-Through Entities

For pass-through entities, such as LLCs, LLPs, and S corporations, the entity will generally need to file a state income tax return and the owners would report the income and pay any related income taxes on their individual income tax returns for the state(s). The reportable net income and other separately stated items on the individual owner's state Schedule K-1, such as charitable contributions and capital gains or losses, may differ from those on the federal return.

Local Income Tax Returns

Some localities require that business entities file income tax returns. This is not the norm, as most counties and cities receive their revenues from other sources, such as business licenses, property taxes, sales and use taxes.

Occupational Taxes

Many local income taxes take the form of occupational taxes. This tax may be withheld from employees, paid solely by the employer, or paid by both the employee and the employer. The taxes, including amounts withheld from the employee paychecks, are remitted by the organization to the city or county on a monthly, quarterly, or annual basis.

The recordkeeping can get complicated. For example, some localities allow an exclusion for income earned outside of the city or county limits. Time spent working at a satellite clinic outside the city limits may not be subject to the main location's occupational tax, may be subject to an occupational tax in the satellite clinic's city, or may not be subject to an occupational tax. In addition, some localities have different tax rates for residents and nonresidents. When employees change addresses, it could affect their tax rate.

State Business and Occupational Taxes

Some states, such as Washington, West Virginia, and Ohio, assess a business and occupational tax, sometimes referred to as a B&O tax. These taxes are covered directly below under gross receipts tax.

Gross Receipts Tax

Several states assess a gross receipts tax on businesses. The tax is based upon gross receipts, rather than taxable (net) income where the practice computes its tax after deducting expenses. States with a gross receipts tax have different methodologies, including one rate for all businesses, different rates for different industries, or graduated rates depending upon amount of gross receipts.

Advocates of gross receipts tax point to the fact that they are easier to administer than the income tax, which can involve complex calculations. Opponents claim that they are unfair, citing the fact that different businesses have different cost structures. In fact, in some cases businesses that suffer losses must still pay this tax.

The gross receipts tax can be incurred instead of or in addition to an income tax. States that currently assess a gross receipts tax instead of an income tax include:

- Nevada
- Ohio
- Texas
- Washington

States that currently assess BOTH a gross receipts tax AND an income tax include:

- Delaware
- Oregon

The following states currently assess NEITHER an income tax nor a gross receipts tax:

- South Dakota
- Wyoming

Taxes That May Be Similar to Gross Receipts Tax

Many business licenses, while not called a "gross receipts tax," are often based upon gross receipts. See the upcoming section on business licenses.

Sales taxes can act in a similar fashion to gross receipts taxes; however, sales taxes are generally structured to exclude certain business-to-business transactions, such as wholesaler to retailer, so as to avoid tax pyramiding or imposing a tax on the same economic value multiple times in the production cycle. See the upcoming Sales Tax section.

Property Taxes

State, county, and city governments assess property taxes on real property, personal property, and intangible property. Taxes on real and personal property are a particularly important source of revenue for local governments and are often referred to as "ad valorem" taxes from the Latin "according to value," because the amount of tax is based upon the value of the item being taxed.

Real Property

If a practice owns real estate, it will most likely pay real estate taxes. An exception might be if the practice were part of a charitable organization that was exempt from these taxes. The tax rate is based upon the assessed value of the property multiplied by the millage, or tax rate. In most areas, it is common for the county to collect these taxes on behalf of the state, county, and city, thus reducing the number of tax bills the practice will receive. In some situations, taxes may be billed separately; for example, in New York state, the school district tax bills are sent separately from the county and town taxes.

The practice will not generally need to file a return to receive this tax bill. The state or local taxing authority will typically send it based upon property records (deeds and sales records) maintained by the county.

Personal Property Tax

This tax is based upon the value of personal property owned by the business. Examples of the items taxed include office furniture, computer equipment and peripherals, and office machines. Sometimes, inventory, leasehold improvements, and/or computer software will be included, depending upon the rules promulgated by the taxing authority. The practice will probably need to file a return or other report listing the personal property with the taxing authority (usually the county) on an annual basis. The information required is similar to the information on the practice's depreciation schedule. Outside accounting firms often prepare this return for smaller practices.

Some states, counties, and municipalities assess an annual ad valorem tax on motor vehicles. This tax is paid when the car tag or license plate is purchased or renewed each year. So, if a practice owns motor vehicle(s), it may pay these taxes. Because lessors often require that the lessee pay these taxes, practices with leased vehicles may also be liable for personal property or ad valorem taxes on these vehicles. Ordinarily, the practice will not file a return for this tax, as the governmental unit (usually the county) will send a bill based upon the vehicle's title. The personal property tax on motor vehicles is in addition to any sales or use tax paid when the practice purchases a vehicle.

Intangibles Tax

These are taxes based upon either the value of or income from intangibles such as securities (stocks, bonds), copyrights, patents, life insurance, and partnership interest held by an organization or individual.

Kansas has an intangibles tax applicable to both corporation and individuals that is assessed on gross earnings received from property such as savings accounts, stocks, bonds, accounts receivable, and mortgages. The rate varies by location, but for most localities it is 2.25%.

Florida has an intangibles tax where businesses must still pay taxes on (1) the value of intangible property secured by mortgage deeds or other liens on certain property and (2) when a taxpayer leases property owned by the government to a nongovernmental entity.

At present, state intangible taxes are not a widespread method of taxation.

Overview of Payroll Taxes

Payroll taxes are those taxes paid based on employee payroll. First, the practice must submit a withholding for federal and, in many cases, state income tax, based on the employee representations on IRS form W-4 and the related state form, if applicable. Both Social Security and Medicare tax liabilities are paid 50% by the employer and 50% by the employee, with the employee amount deducted from employee pay along with the withholding for federal and state income tax.

Employers are also subject to state and federal unemployment taxes. Some states also impose unemployment, disability insurance, or similar taxes on employees.

Self-Employment Taxes

Self-employment taxes are Social Security and Medicare taxes paid by self-employed individuals. The taxes are double the amount withheld from employees; since the self-employed are basically both employer and employee, they pay the taxes for both. These are paid with the self-employed person's individual income tax return and should be included in the estimated tax payments made by the individual. The self-employed tax rate is 15.3% of self-employed income, up to the Social Security wage limit ($137,700 in 2020) and 2.9% of wages over the Social Security wage limit. The self-employed person may also be liable for the additional 0.9% Medicare tax assessed on earnings over a certain amount.

Because these are taxes paid by an individual, they are not generally paid by practices. Healthcare executives need to be aware of the role of the self-employment taxes in two situations:

- The owner physicians in sole proprietorships and partnerships will be liable for self-employment taxes on their personal return, in addition to the income taxes. This can significantly increase the amount of estimated taxes these owners will need to pay. Thus, these owners will often plan to take distributions from the practice to cover the quarterly tax payments shortly before these are due. It is important to make sure to consider this outlay in the entity's cash budgets and projections. The physicians' outside accountant will often make these calculations and provide the related payment instructions.
- If the practice hires independent contractors, the hourly rate may be higher than what the contractor would make as an employee, because the contractor, rather than the practice, is liable for the payroll taxes. The contractor would also be responsible for health insurance, other benefits, and supplies, which can significantly increase the rate per hour as compared to an employee.

Other Taxes

Excise Taxes

Excise taxes are based taxes on consumption and levied on specific goods, services, and activities. They can be either a per unit tax (such as the per gallon tax on gasoline) or a percentage of price (such as the airline ticket tax). Generally, excise taxes are collected from producers or wholesalers, and are embedded in the price paid by final consumers.

Although the excise taxes that most frequently come to mind are those association with gas, diesel, airline tickets, tobacco and firearms, some healthcare products and services are also subject to excise taxes. Many of these were part of the Affordable Care Act:

- Annual fees on health insurance providers, according to their market share. *Note:* This has been appealed for 2021 and beyond.
- Annual fees on manufacturers and importers of branded prescription drugs.
- A 10% tax on indoor tanning services.

Sales Tax

State and local entities impose a sales tax on the sale of goods and/or services. The liability occurs at the point of sale, with the seller being responsible for reporting and submitting the tax to the government. Sales taxes are an important source of revenue for many state and local governments. Some medical practices may be required to collect and remit sales tax on sales of goods and/or services. Most medical practices will need to pay sales tax to vendors on certain purchases. Some of the taxable goods and services may be online sales or purchases.

Practices that sell items such as skin care products, orthopedic devices, and other tangible property must frequently, but not always, collect sales tax from patients/customers on these sales (be sure to check state and local laws). The practice will also be responsible for reporting the taxes to the applicable state and local governments. Although services by the practice's providers are not usually subject to sales taxes, in some states they may be.

Practices that find they are responsible for collecting and remitting sales tax need to ensure that they file the appropriate tax forms and pay the related tax on a timely basis. Usually, this is monthly. Penalties can be expensive.

Most practices will pay sales tax on purchases from vendors, especially when purchasing tangible property. In some states and localities, they may be required to pay sales tax on purchased services. The states of Hawaii, New Mexico, and South Dakota levy sales taxes on accounting services.

The individual responsible for accounts payable for the practice needs to ensure that sales tax is properly charged and that the rates are correct. For example, it is not unusual for neighboring municipalities in urban areas, which might have confusing boundaries, to have different sales tax rates. The borders between municipalities and unincorporated areas in both urban and rural areas can often be confusing, resulting in being charged the wrong amount by a vendor. With a major vendor, that 1% or 2% difference can create a large liability over several years.

The rules governing what is subject to sales tax and the applicable rates vary. One area that varies more than most is software. The states have differing tax methods depending upon whether it is canned software, customized software, downloaded software, loaded from a disc, etc. Mistakes could be expensive in the case of large software purchases, such as Electronic Health Record (EHR), practice management, interfaces, or Laboratory Information System (LIS) software. And the services covered by sales taxes can change. For example, in Texas, medical practices may soon need to pay sales tax on services they receive from outside billing companies. It's vital that the healthcare executive stay abreast of changes affecting their locality.

Generally, a practice should not be charged sales tax on inventory purchased for resale. You may need to provide a tax-exempt number (obtained from your state sales tax agency) to the seller for their records.

A practice that is affiliated with a not-for-profit entity may be exempt from sales tax. You will need to provide your tax-exempt number or certificate to your vendors.

Practices that conduct business over the internet, whether selling or purchasing, will need to be aware of the applicable sales tax rules and regulations. If the practice sells goods (or maybe even medical services) over the internet, it will need to collect and remit sales taxes if it has a nexus in the state. Usually, this means that the practice is registered to do business, or should be registered to do business, in a state. Practices with questions as to whether they have a nexus in state should consult their tax attorney.

When a practice purchases goods or services online, it may or may not be charged sales tax, depending upon whether the vendor believes it has a nexus in the practice's state. If a practice is not charged sales tax on an out-of-state purchase, it may be liable for use tax.

Use taxes apply when sales tax would normally apply but was not charged or collected. For example, a practice might owe use tax if it purchased equipment on which it did not pay sales tax from an out-of-state vendor. These sales may or may not be online sales. The practice would need to ensure that it filed the appropriate use tax forms and paid the related amounts with the applicable state and local governments.

Business Licenses

Business licenses differ from professional licenses in that professional licenses are permits from the state licensing board to practice a profession that requires a demonstrated level of skill and expertise, such as a medical license required for physicians, physician assistants, nurse practitioners, and many other fields. A business license is a local registration that allows a business (including a physician practice) to operate in a specific state, county, or municipality. A practice will most likely need both professional licenses for its professionals and business licenses at the state, county, and/or city level.

Practices operating in multiple locations will most likely need multiple business licenses, especially if the locations are in different municipalities. Separate business licenses may be required for different locations in the same state or municipality. Some localities require a business license for outside businesses that do business in their jurisdiction, while other do not.

The method for computing the cost of the business license and the related rates varies widely among states and municipalities. In addition, the same governmental entity will probably have different license fee methodologies for different types of businesses. The license may be based upon gross receipts, a flat fee, payroll, or a combination of these methods, or some other method. For example, a physician practice may purchase a business license for its primary location based upon a percentage of gross receipts. It might purchase another business license for a satellite location based upon a fixed amount from a sliding scale of gross receipts. It may pay a business license based upon gross payroll for a business office in another location at which no patients are seen.

The practice will need to monitor its state and local license laws and ensure compliance. Keeping a calendar of when these licenses are due is important, as late penalties can be expensive. The practice's accountant is usually a good resource for business license matters.

Franchise Taxes

States charge fees to incorporate or register to do business in that state ("State A"). The initial return is due when the business is either incorporated in State A (a "domestic" corporation or business) or is incorporated in another state ("State B") and begins doing business in State A. (The business incorporated in State B is considered a "foreign" corporation in State A.) The practice will then need to file annual franchise tax returns if it continues to do business in that state or remains incorporated in its home state.

The form may vary based upon the type of entity and whether the entity is organized in that state (domestic) or another state (foreign). Corporations, partnerships, and limited liability entities are generally subject to this tax, while proprietorships are not.

The method of computing the tax varies by state, but the value of the entity's capital is often an important part of the computation.

Some states have a privilege tax (for the "privilege" of doing business in their state) that functions like a franchise tax.

Some states require entities operating within their state to file an annual report. This often lists the business' official address, its officers, and their contact information. This may be part of or combined with the filing of the franchise tax or privilege tax.

Tax Management

The practice should establish clear procedures for managing all tax issues. The practice's chief financial officer (or chief accountant, if there isn't a CFO) should provide oversight and direction to assure that all procedures are followed and that taxes are paid on time. In larger practices, some of these duties can be delegated to a staff accountant.

Most outside accounting firms include tax professionals in their practice or have access to one. Your practice will likely need their expertise from time to time.

If your practice outsources financial operations, make sure that tax services are included in the agreement.

SAMPLE QUESTIONS

1. **Which entity type can have an "unreasonable compensation" issue?**

   A. Partnership

   B. Sole proprietorship

   C. C corporation

   D. Limited liability entity (partnership or corporation)

2. **In general, for which organization type are taxes paid by the entity (as opposed to the owners)?**

   A. Partnership

   B. Sole proprietorship

   C. S corporation

   D. C corporation

Answers: 1-C, 2-D

FINANCIAL MANAGEMENT QUIZ

1. **Arranging for a line of credit from a bank or other lending institution is a good way to prepare for:**

   A. Paying for end-of-year bonuses

   B. Investing in mutual funds

   C. A temporary cash shortfall

   D. Making a major capital expenditure

2. **What is stockholder's equity?**

   A. The amount that shareholders have contributed to the medical practice

   B. The amount that the practice can be sold for, after all debts are paid

   C. The difference between assets and liabilities on the balance sheet

   D. The difference between revenues and expenses on the income statement

3. **What is a major benefit of budgets?**

   A. They communicate actual financial performance to outside stakeholders

   B. They require managers to plan in an organized fashion

   C. They provide long-term estimates of practice revenue and expense

   D. They document actual revenue and expenses over time

4. **The gross collection ratio is defined as cash collections for a period divided by:**

   A. Gross charges for the period

   B. Adjustments for the period

   C. Total patient receipts for the period

   D. Ending accounts receivable balance for the period

5. What entity is legally responsible for ensuring that employee payroll taxes are paid?

A. The employee

B. The federal Internal Revenue Service

C. The employer

D. The state's Department of Labor

ANSWERS

1-C. A line of credit from a bank is considered a form of short-term credit. It is most commonly used to finance ongoing working capital when a business needs to shore up its short-term cash flow.[13]

2-C. Depending on the legal structure of an organization, owner's equity may include contributed capital, undistributed earnings, different classes of stock, donated capital, or retained earnings. In general, stockholder's equity represents the difference between assets and liabilities on the balance sheet.[14]

3-B. The major benefit of budgets is that they require managers to plan in an organized and concentrated way. Budgets are short-range targets expressed in financial terms. The process demands that the medical group set aside a specific time each year to plan and that the plans be built on already-established goals and objectives.[15]

4-A. This ratio indicates the fee-for-service collection margin for the group. The gross collection margin is the amount of actual revenue collected as a percentage of the practice's gross charges. This ratio is used to estimate the amount of services that must be provided to patients to achieve a particular level of revenue for the group. It is also useful for projecting future cash flows based on recent charges.[16]

5-C. By law, the employer is ultimately responsible for ensuring that payroll has been processed accurately and that taxes have been filed appropriately.

Notes

1. Deborah Walker Keegan and Elizabeth W. Woodcock, *The Physician Billing Process: 12 Potholes to Avoid on the Road to Getting Paid*, 3rd ed. (Englewood, CO: Medical Group Management Association, 2016), 102.
2. American Academy of Family Physicians, "Your Revenue Cycle: Denial Rate," aafp.org.
3. David N. Gans, "The High Cost of Dealing with Insurance," *MGMA Connexion* 10, no. 1 (2010), 25-26.
4. Nancy Enos, "Choosing Financial Systems for Medical Group Practices," in *Financial Management for Medical Groups: A Resource for New and Experienced Managers*, 3rd ed. (Englewood, CO: Medical Group Management Association, 2014), 90-91.
5. Ibid, 89.
6. Patrick Dougherty, "Pros and Cons of Outsourcing Medical Billing," M-Scribe.com, Oct. 12, 2017, https://www.m-scribe.com/blog/pros-and-cons-of-outscourcing-medical-billing.
7. *Financial Management for Medical Groups: A Resource for New and Experienced Managers*, 3rd ed. (Englewood, CO: MGMA, 2014), 232, exhibit 8.6.
8. Charles T. Horngren, Srikant M. Datar, and George Foster, *Cost Accounting: A Managerial Emphasis* (Upper Saddle River, NJ: Prentice Hall, 2002), 178.

9. Daniel Liberto, "Chart of Accounts (COA)", Investopedia, Aug. 21, 2020, https://www.investopedia.com/terms/c/chart-of-accounts.asp.
10. "Generally Accepted Auditing Standards," American Institute of Certified Public Accountants (AICPA), page 871, modified November 2006, www.aicpa.org/Research/Standards/AuditAttest/DownloadableDocuments/AU-00150.pdf.
11. Ibid, 871-872.
12. "Chart of Entity Comparison," National Association of Tax Professionals, 2010, http://cpa-services.com/Special%20Articles/chart_of_entity_comparison.pdf.
13. American Express Company, "Line of Credit Basics," *New York Times* (2002), www.nytimes.com/ref/open/finance/OPEN-CREDIT-BASICS.html.
14. "Glossary of Terms Used in Medical Practice Management," Medical Group Management Association, www.mgma.com/WorkArea/DownloadAsset.aspx?id=8688.
15. *Medical Practice Management, Body of Knowledge Review Series: Financial Management, 3rd Edition*, Volume 2 (Englewood, CO: MGMA, 2015), 202.
16. Lee Ann Webster, "Reporting Financial Reports" in *Financial Management for Medical Groups: A Resource for New and Experienced Managers*, 3rd ed. (Englewood, CO: Medical Group Management Association, 2014), 149.

Chapter 3

Human Resource Management

Human resource management involves an effective staffing strategy that includes staff recruitment and retention, training, a performance evaluation process, a personal commitment to enhancing your own knowledge base, and compliance with employment laws.

In this chapter, we will explore the fundamentals of:

1. Clinical and Nonclinical Staffing Plans
2. Clinical and Nonclinical Staff Recruitment
3. Labor Relations and Employment Law (Federal and State)
4. Staff Compensation and Benefit Plans
5. Talent Management
6. Employee Engagement

TASK 1: CLINICAL AND NONCLINICAL STAFFING PLANS

1.1 Staffing Needs Assessment

KEY TERMS

Staffing plan: A staffing plan is part of the overall business plan focused on providing appropriate employees to meet the needs of the practice.

Staffing: The function within an organization responsible for recruiting, screening, and selecting employees. This function may also be responsible for other areas of employment, such as orientation, training, retention, and termination of staff.

Creating a staffing plan is part of business planning. Strategic planning and workforce planning must be aligned for success, and the staffing plan is one piece of an overall business plan. The staffing plan will need to be updated as the business shifts, grows, or contracts and attains or proposes new business goals.

Up to 80% of a medical practice's budget may be focused on staffing, creating huge challenges for the healthcare executive to provide qualified, well-trained staff members at a competitive wage. A healthcare executive should consider how overtime, shift differential pay, and employee status (part-time versus full-time) affect the bottom line in short- and long-term budgets. In order to create the overall budget, the practice should complete a staffing needs assessment.

In order to do this, the executive and the leadership team should consider the overall staffing strategy, the number of patients being served, and the future growth of the practice. Consider how the practice could be run more efficiently, the best staffing mix, and the overall goals for the practice. To conduct a thorough staffing needs assessment, the executive must have a thorough knowledge of growth, contraction, and the staffing mix.

Each healthcare executive needs to determine appropriate staffing levels for the practice, depending on the specialty, additional services provided by the practice, physicians' needs, workflow, and other characteristics. There are a number of variables that affect the staffing plan.

1.2 Position Descriptions

KEY TERMS

Position description: A job description tailored for one specific title.

Job specifications: All the details of a job, including knowledge, skills, and abilities needed.

Job descriptions: A list of the tasks, duties, and responsibilities.

Many terms are used for job descriptions: *position descriptions*, *job specifications*, and of course, *job descriptions*. Typically, a job description encompasses all of these and is the term used here.

Complete, current, and detailed job descriptions help new staff members understand their jobs and remind existing employees what is expected of them. They guide employee selection and placement, help assess training and development needs, and serve as the foundation for performance standards. Formal job descriptions also protect organizations from charges of discrimination because they clearly detail what staff members must be able to do as required by the ADA.

The creation of job descriptions and classifications for the practice is a multifaceted process. First, the types of jobs currently needed and those needed in the future are identified based on the strategic plan of the practice. Next, each job is analyzed according to its vital components — the what, why, and how of the job. Finally, each job's responsibilities, the qualifications needed by the job holder, and relationships to other staff members are described. This allows the healthcare executive to classify the jobs into categories and to move to the next steps of evaluating job value to determine compensation rates.

Job Description Basics

- Reporting structure
- Role qualifications
- Physical demands and essential functions of the job
- Work environment description

SAMPLE QUESTIONS

1. When creating a staffing plan, what information should be considered?

A. Community budget

B. Practice contraction rate

C. Practice budget

D. Competition's staffing pattern

2. Job descriptions should include:

A. Company benefits

B. Marriage status of the applicant

C. Physical demands and essential functions

D. Company rules and policies

Answers: 1-C, 2-C

TASK 2: CLINICAL AND NONCLINICAL STAFF RECRUITMENT

2.1 Recruitment Activities

Recruitment activities are varied and span many types these days. No longer can practices simply place an ad in a newspaper. The best methods of recruitment for your practice may mean using a variety of methods, such as providing recruitment or referral bonuses, using word of mouth and current employees, posting job descriptions on social media and with professional organizations, as well as placing ads online with services such as Indeed or ZipRecruiter.

KEY TERMS

Employment practice: Any recruitment, hiring, selection, transfer or promotion policy, or any benefit provision or other function of the employer's process that operates as an analysis or screening device.

Recruitment: The practice of soliciting and actively seeking applicants to fill recently vacated or newly created positions, using a variety of methods (i.e., internal job postings, advertising in newspapers or electronic job boards or websites, using search firms, or listing positions with trade and professional associations).

Selection process: Any step, combination of steps, or procedure used as a basis for any employment decision, including, but not limited to, informal or casual interviews, application forms, paper and pencil tests, performance tests, training programs, probationary periods, and physical, education, and work experience requirements, as well as the decision-making process used in determining whether or not to hire or promote.

Social media advertising: Recruitment via social media, such as Facebook, Instagram, Twitter, LinkedIn, etc. Most job seekers rely on their own friend groups and professional networks to search for a job.

Search firms/agencies: A search firm is a professional service company hired by the medical practice to help attract, hire, and develop staff members who will hold jobs that are key to achieving the medical practice's goals and objectives. The service is paid for by the medical practice, not by the hired person. Job candidates are presented to the medical group by the search firm based on employer-specified requirements.

2.2 Interviewing

Interviewing is the opportunity for the organization to meet with job applicants and to assess the "fit" for the position. The purpose of the interview is to meet face-to-face to evaluate the skill set of the applicant to determine if the applicant's knowledge and experience matches with the practice's needs. An interview is an excellent opportunity to learn about the applicant's work history and technical job skills as well as to determine personal characteristics to assess the relationship between the potential employee and the practice.

KEY TERMS

Phone or virtual interviews: Phone or virtual interviews allow a pre-screening opportunity to confirm resume or application details.

Job-specific interviews: This is a type of interview that assesses whether the candidate is able to perform the duties of the job according to the skills required. The questions will be specific to the role.

Open-ended questions: Open-ended questions require more than just a "yes" or "no" answer. They encourage candidates to discuss issues and share information about their background, experience, skills, and abilities, so the employer can determine whether the candidate will be a good fit for the position.

Behavior-based questions: Behavior-based interviews present candidates with scenarios and ask how they would respond to those situations.

2.3 Pre-Employment and Onboarding Activities

KEY TERMS

Onboarding: The process by which the organization introduces an employee to the company's culture to help them become a viable member of the team. This process varies in length by company.

Criminal background check: A review of an applicant's criminal history, conducted with consent, post-offer. Check with your state's laws for the number of years you're allowed to review. This is a highly regulated process, and a policy should be reviewed for legal requirements.

Health examination: A health examination to determine if the applicant can meet the essential functions of the position. This is an exam that is conducted confidentially and post-offer.

Drug screening: A screening for illicit drug use after the job offer has been made. Employers who choose to use drug tests should test all applicants as a condition of employment. Results of all drug screenings should be maintained in confidential files with the employee's health file, separate from the personnel file.

The pre-employment phase and various onboarding activities are an essential part of bringing a new employee into the organization. Once the candidate has agreed to the position, the pre-employment phase begins. This involves everything from testing, background checks, health information, and more. Pre-employment should be a timely and thorough process that is consistent, no matter the position or the person. This phase should result in a better new hire and a better hiring process overall, eliminating any hiring bias or unfair advantages as long as the process is the same for everyone. This phase reviews job fit, skill fit, and pre-employment testing to confirm the candidate is "right" for the practice.

Onboarding is the process of bringing new employees into the organization by providing information, training, mentoring, and coaching during their first six to 12 months of employment. It helps new employees more quickly contribute to the organization, increases their comfort level, reinforces their decision to join the organization, enhances productivity, and encourages employee commitment, engagement, and retention. Research has also demonstrated that, more than traditional orientation programs, onboarding reduces stress and the chance of employees quitting soon after starting.

Onboarding and new employee orientation programs help employees develop a self-identity and a team spirit, which contribute to healthy attitudes toward the medical group and can lower absenteeism and employee turnover. They are an effective way to communicate that the medical practice demands full effort from its employees to maximize productivity and the quality of services, and also that the practice values and respects its employees. These programs also inform new hires about the practice's policy prohibiting unlawful discrimination and harassment.

Conduct official background checks after an employment offer and prior to the employee's first day of work to verify that the employee doesn't have any undisclosed criminal history. An employment offer can be made contingent on successful results of a background or reference check.

Background investigations and reference checks are the principal means by which employers actively check into the backgrounds of potential hires. Each can involve both verifying information provided by applicants and ascertaining pertinent information not provided by applicants themselves. A background investigation generally involves screening out persons who are not qualified because of criminal convictions, poor driving records, poor credit history, or misrepresentations on resumes or application forms about education or prior work history.

SAMPLE QUESTIONS

1. **What should be considered when interviewing potential staff members?**

   A. Request information about personal life

   B. Skill set review pertinent to position applying

   C. Number of full-time-equivalent staff to full-time-equivalent physicians

   D. Number of full-time-equivalent primary care physicians to full-time-equivalent specialty physicians

2. **An interview is effective if it includes:**

   A. Reading the job description to the candidate

   B. Asking yes-or-no questions

   C. A combination of interview techniques

   D. Only the interviewer and candidate

Answers: 1-B, 2-C

TASK 3: LABOR RELATIONS AND EMPLOYMENT LAW (FEDERAL AND STATE)

State and federal laws require employers to create and maintain certain employment-related records. Labor laws allow employees the right to unionize and to participate in strikes, picketing, and lockouts to have their demands met. The healthcare executive's human resource function, along with legal counsel, can help the medical group address local union activity, organizing tactics and targets, early warning signs of union involvement, lawful employer countermeasures, effective personnel policies and practices, and the employer's legal rights in dealing with a union.

3.1 Regulatory Compliance

Regulatory compliance is the practice's efforts to assure they are complying with all appropriate and relevant laws, regulations and directives set forth by the local, state and federal government. These regulations and laws differ from state to state, and local counties and cities as well.

KEY TERMS

The key terms presented below are federal rules that must be followed throughout the country regardless of local or state rules. Your state or local ordinance may have added measures to these rules. Please check with your appropriate local and state regulators to determine local requirements.

FMLA: The Family and Medical Leave Act (FMLA) requires covered employers to provide up to 12 weeks of unpaid, job-protected leave to eligible employees for certain family and medical reasons. Medical practice employees are eligible if they have worked for the medical practice for more than one year, for 1,250 hours over the previous 12 months, and if there are at least 50 employees within the medical group within 75 miles of the practice's main office (some employees may work offsite or at satellite clinics, but these must be within a 75-mile radius).

ADA - Americans with Disabilities Act of 1990: The Americans with Disabilities Act (ADA) prohibits private employers, state and local governments, employment agencies, and labor unions from discriminating against qualified individuals with disabilities in job application procedures, hiring, firing, advancement, compensation, job training, and other aspects of employment. The ADA covers employers with 15 or more employees. An individual with a disability, defined as a protected individual, is a person who has a physical or mental impairment that substantially limits one or more major life activities, has a record of such impairment, or is regarded as having such impairment.

continued on next page

Civil Rights: *Title VII of the Civil Rights Act of 1964*: Under Title VII and corresponding EEOC regulations, an employer who maintains employment records (any records having to do with hiring, transfer, demotion, promotion, layoff, termination, rates of pay, and selection for training programs) must keep the records for a period of one year from the date the records were made or one year from the date of the personnel action, whichever is longer.

ACA: The Patient Protection and Affordable Care Act (ACA), and the Health Care and Education Reconciliation Act amending the ACA were signed into law on March 23 and 30, 2010, respectively. Employers with more than 50 employees face tax penalties if they do not provide all full-time employees with affordable healthcare coverage.

EEOC - Equal Employment Opportunity Commission: The EEOC is the government agency with significant effect on employment law. It regulates and enforces federal Equal Employment Opportunity (EEO) laws to prevent discriminatory practices.

ADEA - Age Discrimination in Employment Act of 1967 (ADEA): Under the ADEA, a covered employer must keep records on each employee, which include name, date of birth, address, occupation, rate of pay, and weekly compensation. These records must be kept for at least three years.

OSHA - Occupational Safety and Health Administration: The Occupational Safety and Health Act of 1970 created the Occupational Safety and Health Administration (OSHA). OSHA requires employers with more than 10 employees to keep a record of serious work-related injuries and illnesses.

NLRA/NLRB - National Labor Relations Act: The Wagner Act of 1935, otherwise known as the National Labor Relations Act (NLRA), was passed to protect employees' rights to unionize. The National Labor Relations Board (NLRB) was created to implement and enforce the NLRA.

Pregnancy Discrimination Act: The Pregnancy Discrimination Act of 1978 amended the Civil Rights Act, stating that discrimination on the basis of pregnancy, childbirth, or related medical conditions constitutes unlawful sex discrimination under Title VII.

Immigration Reform and Control Act of 1986: Employers are required to have all new employees complete the I-9 form to verify that they are eligible to work in the United States. Employers must keep I-9 forms for either three years or one year after termination, whichever is longer. Some states also have laws related to verification of work eligibility that may contain additional recordkeeping requirements.

Please note: Throughout the year, there may be changes to various laws or regulations. It is important to your practice to check with the local, state and federal government agencies for any updates or changes throughout the year.

3.2 Company Policies and Procedures

Company policies and procedures are a fundamental part of creating an organization that clearly communicates with its employees. The medical practice needs to communicate its policies, procedures, employee benefits, management and employee responsibilities, and other essential information to all employees. A good way to provide this information is by creating an employee handbook. Use clear and precise language, including terminology, when developing policies and procedures. Solicit your legal counsel or an appropriate consultant to review the language in all of your medical practice's policies.

The employee handbook is one of the most important communication tools for both the employer and its employees. It can be used as a marketing and branding tool for current and prospective employees. It is an important management tool and resource document, and it contains employment legal documentation.

SAMPLE QUESTIONS

1. **Which of the following is considered employment law?**
   A. Benefits summary
   B. Grievance Policy and Procedure
   C. Motor Vehicle Law
   D. National Labor Relations Act

2. **Company policies should include:**
   A. Personal information about the operators
   B. Written information
   C. Practice financials
   D. Community feedback

Answers: 1-D, 2-B

TASK 4: STAFF COMPENSATION AND BENEFIT PLANS

Formal employee benefits may include medical, dental, and vision plans, short- and long-term disability insurance, life insurance, pension plan, savings and investment plans, unemployment insurance, and staff members' compensation premiums, among others. These benefits usually have a shared cost between the employer and employee, based on a certain percentage.

KEY TERMS

Paid time off (PTO): Some employers are moving to a flexible program of paid time off (PTO) that combines time off for sick leave, vacation, holidays, and jury duty into one pool.

Recruitment bonus: Employees may be provided with a recruitment, signing, or referral bonus if a person is referred to the medical practice, accepts the position, and stays in the position for a certain period of time.

Eligibility: Benefit plans can be established for certain employee types and classes of employees. A medical practice can define the difference between full-time and part-time employment for benefit purposes.

Defined-benefit plans: Include pension and annuity plans that offer a specific retirement benefit to employees, such as a monthly payment based on prior employee wages and years of service.

Defined-contribution plan: A company retirement plan, such as a 401(k) or 403(b) plan, in which the employee elects to defer some amount of their salary into the plan and bears the investment risk. The employer may provide some level of contribution to these plans as well.

Employer-directed plan: A retirement account in which the employer makes investment decisions.

401(k) and 403(b): Retirements savings into which employees may contribute a pretax, fixed amount or some percentage of their income on an annual basis. The employer may provide some level of contribution to these plans as well.

Pension plan: A qualified retirement plan set up by a corporation, labor union, government, or other organization for its employees. A business could offer a profit-sharing plan, a stock bonus plan, an employee stock ownership plan, a thrift plan, a target benefit plan, a money purchase pension plan, or a defined benefit plan.

Profit-sharing plan: An arrangement in which an employer shares some of its profits with its employees. The compensation can be stocks, bonds, or cash, and can be immediate or deferred until retirement. Profit sharing allows for changing contributions each year. Contributions are determined by a formula to allocate the overall contribution and

continued on next page

distribution of accumulated funds after the retirement age. Contributions and earnings can currently grow tax-deferred until withdrawal.

Self-directed plan: A retirement account in which an employee makes their own decisions about which stocks, bonds, and mutual funds to buy.

4.1 Benefit Selections

The types of insurance that may be offered are generally health and/or life.

Access to health insurance coverage is a key benefit for a medical practice. Employees may seek employment based on whether the employer offers health insurance. While it might be the case that some smaller medical practices do not offer health insurance to their employees, most larger practices have to offer health insurance to competitively recruit and retain employees. In addition to basic health insurance, additional specific health-related insurance may include the following:

- Charitable matching contributions
- Child care or elder care
- Consolidated Omnibus Budget Reconciliation Act of 1985
- Dental, vision, and hearing insurance
- Financial planning or counseling
- Housing financing assistance
- In-house medical services. As an employee benefit, medical practices may offer access to certain types of medical services within the organization.
- Individual Retirement Accounts (IRA)
- Length of Service awards or gifts
- Life insurance
- Long-term and short-term disability insurance
- Long-term care plans
- Paid time off or vacation/sick/holiday accruals
- Post-employment medical benefits
- Recruitment bonuses
- Retention bonuses
- Retirement benefits

SAMPLE QUESTIONS

1. Employee benefits are:

A. Insurance for the employee's family

B. Financial and nonfinancial rewards and incentives provided to employees in return for employment

C. Overtime, salary, and bonuses

D. Medical insurance and payroll taxes

2. ________ should be considered when determining benefits packages:

A. Staff family makeup

B. Pregnancy leave

C. Recruitment and retention attractiveness

D. Medicaid costs

Answers: 1-B, 2-C

TASK 5: TALENT MANAGEMENT

Talent management is managing the people you have (the talent) and assisting them in their growth, optimizing their aptitudes in order to maintain and succeed in the practice's goals and vision. It's a way to describe how you encourage and assist your staff to become successful in your practice. It all begins with who you hire and continues with how you orient, onboard, and train them, progressing long afterward with career development, conflict resolution, performance management, and evaluations.

KEY TERMS

- **Performance appraisal or evaluation:** A periodic review and assessment of an individual's job performance.
- **Performance-based pay:** A variable pay strategy that pays employees based on their individual performance and contributions, rather than the value of the job they are performing.
- **Performance counseling:** The process of improving employee performance and productivity by providing employees with feedback regarding areas where they are doing well and areas that may require improvement.
- **Performance improvement plan:** A plan implemented by a manager or supervisor that is designed to provide employees with constructive feedback, facilitate discussions between an employee and their supervisor regarding performance-related issues, and outline specific areas of performance requiring improvement.
- **Performance management:** The process of maintaining or improving employee job performance through the use of performance assessment tools, coaching, and counseling, as well as providing continuous feedback.
- **Performance monitoring:** The practice of monitoring employees while they perform their jobs through the use of surveillance cameras or telephone or computer monitoring.
- **Performance standards:** The tasks, functions, or behavioral requirements established by the employer as goals to be accomplished by an employee.
- **Succession planning:** Preparing your practice for changes, fluctuating business models, and any transformations in the future.
- **Staff development:** Providing opportunity for training and advancement for your employees and staff.
- **Training:** The act of sharing information and teaching staff members information for their position.

5.1 Succession Planning

Succession planning, is to a certain degree, not discussed either because healthcare executives or physicians think it is solely about death or retirement, or because they don't really know what it is. In actuality, succession planning involves retaining talented employees, planning for the future, and giving opportunities to those who have potential.

5.2 Staff Development

Practices must provide their employees with ongoing training and professional development. This can be done through internal means (staff meetings, training sessions, etc.) or through external methods (association meetings, consultants, paid training sessions). Continuing education builds a solid foundation of knowledge for employees to better perform their jobs. Every medical group needs its employees to have continuing education updates on safety (e.g., OSHA, universal precautions, fire prevention) and compliance (e.g., HIPAA, correct billing practices), along with updates on technology and regulatory changes (e.g., Medicare, Medicaid, state laws). Continuing education may also be needed to keep an employee licensed or registered in a particular profession, and to improve interpersonal, leadership, or other personal skill sets.

Effective training requires a positive learning environment, quality materials, motivated and incentivized employees, and adult learning models based on the needs of the group being trained. Training sessions must be staffed by trained professionals as opposed to experts in content material, and by people who can teach adults using a variety of teaching methods.

5.3 Staff Training

Training content determination is a multidisciplinary group process. Usually, groups identify more topics and issues than can possibly be covered. Teams can help prioritize topics and the level of detail needed for training, and this, in turn, largely determines the type of training that is pursued.

The variety of training offered in the practice ranges from orientation and onboarding to supervisory and management training, including ongoing development; technical and skills-based training; career development for the employee to create career advancement opportunities; certification; cross-training; and basic introductory training for recent graduates.

Training can be delivered in many ways, such as web-based, streaming formats and webinars, interactive in-person training, role-playing, lectures, group discussions and meetings, books and materials. Training can be completed in-house or it can be outsourced. All trainings should be evaluated for effectiveness in order to create long-standing change. If training is conducted in-house, the practice must train the trainer. The trainer must be knowledgeable and comfortable using adult learning principles.

5.4 Performance Evaluations

The performance management system, which includes performance planning, evaluation, and rating, is a vital component of human resource management. The timing of performance evaluations can be determined by what is the best time for your practice. The most important factors are consistency and regularity, i.e. not skipping years as the business ramps up or slows down. Whatever the policy is on performance evaluations, it needs to be maintained. If deviations must occur, employees should receive a written notice.

Performance evaluations can be used to review the year's progress as well as to help the employee reach individual goals and support practice goals. It is critical that employers have a performance management system that accurately measures and improves employee performance and that is legally defensible. There is a clear link between the successful operation and the effective and efficient performance of its employees. A comprehensive performance management process can help the organization attract and retain highly qualified employees and ensure quality, cost-effective service. As a result, both employee and employer goals are achieved.

The medical group should establish performance expectations at the beginning of an employee's tenure, reinforce them consistently, and reward positive results regularly. Your group should provide a uniform and general framework for performance management, which ensures that employees know what is expected of them and supervisors know how to establish a job-related basis for planning, managing, and evaluating performance.

5.5 Staff Retention

KEY TERMS

Retention: Keeping employees in the practice.

Turnover: The number of employees who leave and must be replaced in a year (e.g., calendar year, fiscal year, etc.).

Finding a way to retain and motivate your top employees increases productivity and profitability. Labor costs are the largest expense in most group practices. Losing qualified and capable employees is costly. Not only is the turnover cost an actual dollar figure, but it also takes a toll on the business to have the position unfilled, requiring other staff members to take on additional responsibilities, which can cause frustration with management. These are unqualified numbers that are difficult to monetize, but possibly more important than the actual turnover costs, which include the process of recruitment, interviewing and onboarding.

Employees leave positions not just for increased salaries. The majority of employees leave because:

- There is discord with current supervisor or manager
- There is little to no career growth
- There is unsatisfactory pay and/or benefits
- The culture is not compatible

When the employment market was more fluid, medical groups regarded retention-related orientation programs as an afterthought of the recruitment function. This often limited a physician orientation to a rote explanation of the rules, compensation, and other company policies necessary to ensure smooth personnel functions. Now, the emphasis in orientation is moving from the end of the recruitment function to the beginning of the retention process.

The challenge today is not only revamping outdated incentive and retention programs and designing new ones, but also continually implementing, managing, and evaluating their results. Successfully implementing these programs can help your group practice retain a more motivated, productive workforce while making a significant contribution to the practice's bottom line.

SAMPLE QUESTIONS

1. **Succession planning is best done:**
   A. When the owner wants to retire
   B. As employees leave the practice
   C. When employees no longer get along
   D. Any time throughout the life of the practice

2. **When designing training programs, the initial item to consider in the development stage is:**
   A. Adult learning principles
   B. Types of training to offer
   C. Needs of the practice
   D. Career advancement for the staff

3. **The ultimate purpose of a performance evaluation is to:**
   A. Review performance over the last year
   B. Share performance information with employee
   C. Enhance the employee's skill set
   D. Explain the goals of the practice

Answers: 1-D, 2-C, 3-B

TASK 6: EMPLOYEE ENGAGEMENT

KEY TERMS

Culture: The beliefs and thought processes of the organization that affect the employees' beliefs about the workplace.

Engagement: How connected the employees feel toward the practice.

Job satisfaction: The level of enjoyment or approval an employee feels in the workplace.

Open-door policy: An expression that indicates a manager encourages employees to feel free to talk with them, signified by literally leaving their office door open, so an employee is comfortable entering the manager's office.

Overall Engagement

Employee engagement is a real issue and challenge in our workforce. Engagement is a philosophy, a commitment, and an attainable goal for your workplace to have. Each and every employee should share the practice's goals, outlook, mission and overall vision, thus affecting every aspect of work. It is a basic and essential consideration for the overall strategy of the business. Engagement begins with who you hire and continues with how you orient, onboard and train, and finishes with how you retain your staff.

Gallup's 2017 *State of the American Workforce* report says that businesses in the top 25% of employee engagement had less turnover and significantly higher profitability, revenues, and percentages of customer loyalty. The correlation between employee engagement and productivity is strong. The Gallup report also states that employees have a "grass is greener" mentality.

Engagement begins by providing your employees with everything they need to do their jobs successfully. Employees should have all the materials and supplies they need within an arm's reach to be as productive as possible. Your supervisors should be sure that new hires have the necessary resources and training to start working in their new positions immediately and to continue their work throughout the year. They should have clear job descriptions outlining their roles within your practice.

Your group practice should clearly communicate to all employees what is expected of them; what the mission, vision, and culture of the group practice are; what the group practice values; and how the group practice measures success. Employees cannot be engaged or productive if they do not know what is expected of them and how they will be evaluated. Your group practice's vision should be shared by all top-level managers, and you should encourage your employees to help the group practice achieve its vision. Employees become motivated and engaged when the rewards they earn truly mean something. Getting to know each of your employees' personality and behavioral traits, and providing employee-specific rewards will increase productivity, engagement, motivation, and retention. Many people want to feel that their skills are being used to the optimal level in their jobs. Managers should be aware of the skills all of their employees have and place them in jobs that optimize those skills. Employees should also be given responsibilities that they find challenging but not overly stressful.

Engagement Measurement and Benchmarking

Taking the pulse of your employees in the hopes to improve employee satisfaction is not just a one-time thing. This is something that can be accomplished daily, weekly, monthly, and, of course, annually. Employees who speak up and share their daily frustrations to managers and leaders are your greatest knowledge base.

Measuring overall job satisfaction can be done in a variety of ways in order to get real feedback from your teams. Whichever way your practice chooses to gather the information, the most important qualities of a meaningful satisfaction survey are asking the right questions and providing confidentiality. If the culture in the past has been retaliatory, or negative behavior has been allowed previously, it will be a challenge to get participation.

In order to dispel myths and combat long-standing beliefs, it is important to have an open dialogue and conversation with employees as a group, as well as in writing, to address the concerns. Discussing the previous issues — the elephant in the room — must take place in order to get worthwhile information.

Satisfaction surveys are an opportunity to have an open conversation and a real dialogue with employees to improve the workplace. Build upon survey results year after year in order to create long-lasting and positive change. If swift change is needed, using two-year look backs is helpful to adjust every year going forward. If extensive changes are necessary, perhaps institute a mid-year survey as well to make sure the practice is meeting its targets.

Employees will feel a sense of ownership and desire to improve the targeted metrics if they are asked to participate in a meaningful way. If employees are asked to participate so the practice has more information, but they don't see rapid effects or changes, it will have the opposite effect and further derail the practice's efforts. If the plan designed for improvement is a multi-year approach, employees need to understand that to maintain motivation.

SAMPLE QUESTIONS

1. **Engagement is:**

   A. Continuing education

   B. Offering rewards and incentives

   C. Relationships in the workplace

   D. Hiring, training, motivating, and retaining top talent

2. **Which is the most common reason group practices lose employees from the practice?**

   A. Supervisors

   B. Salary and benefits

   C. Better opportunities

   D. Peers and coworkers

Answers: 1-D, 2-A

HUMAN RESOURCE MANAGEMENT QUIZ

1. Which is a key component to a post-offer of employment?

A. Healthcare utilization rate

B. Marriage and family history

C. Workers' compensation check

D. Reference check

2. Family Medical Leave Act eligibility states employees must be:

A. Contracted for more than one year

B. Employed one year and worked at least 1,250 hours

C. Employed one year, working part time

D. Eligible for company benefits

3. An I-9 form should be retained along with the following items:

A. Health file

B. No other documents

C. Other I-9 forms

D. Employee personnel file

4. Licensure verification should occur:

A. Upon hire

B. Before an offer is made

C. Upon hire and annually

D. Upon hire, annually, and post-expiration

ANSWERS

1-D. Searching an employee's background for a claim of workers' compensation may be unlawful. If the employee has a claim for an occupational injury, the employer may be entitled to such information. However, prior to any such injury, it may prove difficult to claim necessity for such information.[1]

2-B. Employees who have been employed one year and worked more than 1,250 hours in a year as defined by your policies are eligible for Family Medical Leave under the Family Medical Leave Act governed by the Department of Labor.[2]

3-C. The United States Citizenship and Immigration Services (USCIS) recommends employers to keep the Form I-9 from personnel records to facilitate an inspection request.[3] A best practice is to retain all I-9 forms together in alphabetized order.

4-D. Licensure verification requirements may be subject to your local or state requirements. The best practice is to verify licensure and/or certification upon hire, annually (e.g., during evaluation or one month during the year) and when the licensure has expired and a new license is presented.

Notes

1. *Medical Practice Management, Body of Knowledge Review Series: Human Resource Management, 4th Edition*, Volume 3 (Englewood, CO: MGMA, 2020).
2. "FMLA Frequently Asked Questions," U.S. Department of Labor, https://www.dol.gov/agencies/whd/fmla.
3. "Retention and Storage," U.S. Citizenship and Immigration Services, https://www.uscis.gov/i-9-central/complete-correct-form-i-9/retention-and-storage.

Chapter 4

Transformative Healthcare Delivery

Medical practices employ a variety of strategies to deliver care and compete in a constantly evolving landscape. The key knowledge and tasks covered in this chapter are:

1. Care Models
2. Payment Models
3. Organizational Models
4. Innovation and Emerging Technologies

TASK 1: CARE MODELS

Medical groups can employ a variety of options for managing the care of the patients they serve in order to improve outcomes and offer more patient-friendly solutions. The approaches noted in this chapter will continue to evolve, so it is vital that today's healthcare executives stay informed about the latest developments.

KEY TERMS

Accountable care organization (ACO): Groups of doctors, hospitals, and other healthcare providers, who come together voluntarily to give coordinated high-quality care to the Medicare patients they serve.

Concierge medicine: Arrangement where a patient pays an annual fee or retainer to a primary care physician to ensure adequate time and availability.

continued on next page

Patient-centered medical home (PCMH): A model or philosophy of primary care that is patient-centered, comprehensive, team-based, coordinated, accessible, and focused on quality and safety.

Team-based care: Multiple clinicians working together to treat a patient.

Direct primary care: Patients pay a monthly fee for timely, convenient access to a physician and a limited menu of basic primary care services. Typically, direct primary care doctors do not accept insurance plans.

Health information exchange: Secure aggregators of patient health information from multiple sources.

Advanced directives: Patient-initiated documentation of expectations for end-of-life care, often paired with a living will and durable power of attorney.

Community benefit organization: Charitable organization designed to support community members in need.

Types of Care Models and Their Applications

Independent medical groups and those affiliated with health systems recognize the need to respond to market forces such as consumer demand. Different reimbursement approaches can place some risk on providers. The models described below are considered to be some of the more innovative approaches to organizing the delivery of patient care.

E-Health

The term *e-health* (from electronic health) broadly refers to computer support for healthcare services, though some confine the definition to healthcare services provided over the internet. E-health continues to revolutionize healthcare delivery. It provides new ways to deliver and manage care, and its goals include improving patient access, increasing quality, decreasing cost, and increasing portability of care, among others.

Examples of e-health applications can include:

- Electronic health records: enabling the communication of patient data among different healthcare professionals
- Computerized physician order entry
- E-prescribing: access to prescribing options, printing prescriptions for patients, and electronic transmission of prescriptions from doctors to pharmacists
- Clinical decision support system: provides information electronically about protocols and standards for healthcare professionals to use in diagnosing and treating patients

- Telemedicine: physical and psychological diagnosis and treatment at a distance, including telemonitoring of patients' key diagnostics

Advantages of e-health can include:

- Empowering patients/consumers
- Improving quality using codified evidence-based protocols
- Enabling providers and medical practices to facilitate and streamline the delivery of care

Challenges of e-health can include:

- Learning new technology
- Changing workflow, including standardizing new protocols and processes
- Investing in the cost of technology
- Learning to manage less face-to-face interaction
- Providing resources to sufficiently support ongoing IT platforms

Accountable Care Organization

The Centers for Medicare and Medicaid Services (CMS) defines accountable care organizations (ACOs) as "... groups of doctors, hospitals, and other healthcare providers, who come together voluntarily to give coordinated high-quality care to the Medicare patients they serve. Coordinated care helps ensure that patients, especially the chronically ill, get the right care at the right time, with the goal of avoiding unnecessary duplication of services and preventing medical errors. When an ACO succeeds in both delivering high-quality care and spending healthcare dollars more wisely, it will share in the savings it achieves for the Medicare program."[1] ACOs tie reimbursement to performance on cost and quality metrics and often use capitation as one form of reimbursement. The practice should reference the specific CMS ACO standards if it expects to participate in an ACO.[2]

Patient-Centered Medical Home

The patient-centered medical home (PCMH) can best be described as a model or philosophy of primary care that is patient centered, comprehensive, team-based, coordinated, accessible, and focused on quality and safety. The structure of PCMH encourages providers and care teams to meet patient needs from the simple to the complex, assuring healthcare professionals provide care in the right place, at the right time, and in a manner that best matches patients' needs. It is most often utilized by primary care medical practices (family medicine, internal medicine, OB/GYN, and pediatrics).

The Agency for Healthcare Research and Quality (AHRQ) lists the following attributes[3] of PCMH:

- Patient-centered: A partnership among practitioners, patients, and their families ensures that decisions respect patients' wants, needs, and preferences, and that patients have the education and support they need to make decisions and participate in their own care

- Comprehensive: A team of care providers is wholly accountable for a patient's physical and mental health needs, including prevention and wellness, acute care, and chronic care
- Coordinated: Care is organized across all elements of the broader healthcare system, including specialty care, hospitals, home health, community services, and supports
- Accessible: Patients can access services with shorter wait times, "after hours" care, 24/7 electronic or telephone access, and strong communication through health IT innovations
- Commitment to quality and safety: Clinicians and staff embrace quality improvement efforts to ensure that patients and families make informed decisions about their health

Managing Care

Practices have implemented a variety of strategies to adapt to the multiple stresses put on them by new care delivery and payment models.

Patient Access and Continuity

Professional societies such as the American Association of Family Practitioners (AAFP) have advised their members on how to provide access and continuity to their patients in the medical home. Examples, such as those from the AFFP, include[4] recommendations for patient access.

Patients should have access to providers, including:

- Access 24/7 for urgent needs
  - Timely contact to address urgent needs
  - Patients and clinicians should be able to remotely log in to electronic health records
- Patients should be able to schedule same-day appointments (open-access or advanced-access scheduling). *Note:* The practice should match patient needs and staff resources to decide how best to accommodate patient needs.
- Practices should offer extended hours, including early mornings, evenings, and weekends.
- Practices can offer a variety of electronic connection opportunities, which can include telemedicine, secure messaging, and patient portals.

Panel Management and Patient Continuity

Empanelment is the process of identifying and assigning active patients to clinicians or care teams to establish and maintain patient-clinician relationships.

The empanelment process includes identifying the ideal panel per clinician, developing initial patient panels, refining the panels based on clinician input and ideal panel size, and ongoing panel management. Panels may fluctuate over time due to changes in the practice's panel, as well as the practice's staffing model.

Empanelment enhances care by increasing access, supporting care coordination, and improving continuity, resulting in improved outcomes and lower cost. Creating a meaningful connection between physicians and their patients goes a long way to ensuring that patients receive optimal care.

Care coordination involves organizing and communicating patient care to the entire team involved in their care in order to improve the safety and quality of that care, and to assure patient needs and preferences are accounted for in advance of care delivery.

Team-Based Care

Cognizant of the need for care continuity, team-based care provides the means for multiple clinicians to treat patients by collaborating with each other. Depending upon patient needs, members of the care team can include physicians, nurse practitioners, physician assistants, nurses, and other allied staff such as physical or speech therapists.[5]

In their paper *Implementing Optimal Team-Based Care to Reduce Clinician Burnout*, the authors state, "A team-based model of care strives to meet patient needs and preferences by actively engaging patients as full participants in their care, while encouraging all healthcare professionals to function to the full extent of their education, certification, and experience."[6]

Effective team-based care goes a long way toward improving patient outcomes and patient experience. In addition, the push to value-based care relies upon effective teamwork.

To implement team-based care, practices begin by defining the roles of different care team members, by using member skills at the highest capacity. It is also necessary to create processes for sharing both written and verbal information about the patient, ensuring that each care team member has all the data needed to make informed care decisions.

Population Health Management

Population health management is a team-based approach that focuses on prevention, early intervention, and close partnerships with patients to aggressively manage chronic conditions. Population health management enables a practice to:

- Use data stored in patient registries to identify patients who can benefit from evidence-based chronic or preventive care
- Create and manage plans of care based on patient diseases or conditions
- Support patient self-management
- Monitor progress and recommend changes to care plans supported by functionality in the electronic health record

- Monitor care team performance by tracking patient data and comparing it with both national guidelines and internal benchmarks and expectations

Using the techniques of population health management, physicians and other clinicians can more proactively identify health needs of the practice's patient population and determine how best to meet those needs.[7]

Care Management and Support

Care management and support refers to the protocols used to manage patients whose conditions require more monitoring and management. This approach facilitates improved outcomes and lower cost of care by reducing unnecessary complications.

Once patients are categorized in risk groups, providers use standard protocols to guide care, including monitoring of disease indicators, care coordination among specialists, and collaboration with community resources.

Care Coordination and Care Transitions

Care coordination refers to the communication, activities, and accountability among medical professionals in the care of higher risk patients. Communication includes the sharing of information such as medical history, medication lists, and test results. Care activities may include determining needs, updating plans of care, and connecting patients with resources to augment care. Providers establish accountability by clearly identifying who is responsible for each aspect of the patient's care.

Care coordination often includes the following specific activities:[8]

- Determine and update care management and coordination needs
- Create and update the plan of care
- Exchange information among those accountable for the patient's care
- Facilitate transitions
- Connect with community
- Align resources with patient needs

Performance Measurement and Quality Improvement

Quality improvement refers to establishing a culture of data-driven performance improvement efforts covering clinical quality, efficiency, and patient experience that engages staff and patients, families, and caregivers. Metrics can include common preventive actions such as breast cancer screening, vaccinations, and screening for depression. In addition, these efforts support and enhance care coordination, especially for higher risk patients.

Tracking performance against benchmarks can then be used to identify areas for improvement.

Concierge Medicine and Direct Primary Care

Concierge medicine (also known as retainer medicine) refers to the arrangement where a patient pays an annual fee or retainer to a primary care physician. To ensure adequate time and availability for each patient, doctors agree to limit patient loads. Under these arrangements, patients can still be charged for certain services.

Considered a type of concierge medicine, a direct primary care doctor charges each patient a monthly fee in return for timely, convenient access and a limited menu of basic primary care services. Direct primary care doctors do not accept insurance.

Performance Management

Successful physician practices commit to continuous performance improvement in all aspects of their operation. This is especially critical in care delivery as it impacts the health of the patients, their experience, and the cost of delivering care.

Clinical Processes and Outcomes

Clinical process and outcome efforts look at finding the most effective ways to deliver care with the intent of improving patient health for those with chronic conditions. Initiatives in this area can include setting protocols based on the latest research of how patients are treated for specific conditions.

Clinical Variation Reduction

Closely related to clinical process improvement is the reduction in clinical variation. Using standard care protocols works best if there is regular monitoring of performance against standards. Those tasked with examining the data must work with clinicians to explain variances from prescribed protocols and processes. This provides a means to objectively pursue performance improvement.

Patient Experience

A positive patient experience not only improves satisfaction, but it can also contribute to greater compliance with prescribed treatments. Practices implement regular surveys and other forms of patient feedback, which can help to prioritize initiatives aimed at performance improvement.

Practice Efficiency

Practice efficiency initiatives aspire to improve all processes in the practice with the expectation of lowering the cost of providing care. Routinely polling providers and staff can be a great way to discover opportunities for improvement and cost reduction. One example would be the decision to verify a patient's insurance prior to their visit to assure that the practice can get paid, and collect out-of-pocket payments (co-pays) at the time of the visit.

Population Health Analytics

Population heath refers to the health outcomes of a group of individuals, including the distribution of such outcomes within the group.[9] Physicians can successfully manage what they measure. Population health analytics provide actionable information to reduce risk. Valuable information can include the various demographic profiles (e.g., age and socioeconomic distribution), as well as more clinical measures such as incidence of pre-diabetic conditions.

Practices will need to acquire meaningful data and understand how to use it. Data will come from multiple sources, including the practice EMR, claims data, data from affiliated practices, and hospitals where the physician admits. In addition, many communities and provider groups participate in health information exchanges (HIE), which aggregate the information from multiple sources.

The group should agree on the timing of regular reports, often quarterly. Leadership can set meetings to explore how patients, especially those with chronic conditions, are faring and discuss as a group what can be done, if anything, to improve outcomes.

Strategies to Manage Risk

Payers increasingly expect physicians to take on risk, whether through fixed payments such as a capitation or incentives through paying for value.

Identifying High-Risk Patients

While often small in number, high-risk patients account for a majority of healthcare spending. As a result, early identification and management of this population proves key to improving outcomes and lowering the cost of care. The National Association of Community Health Centers lists four types of risk profiles for patients:[10]

1. Highly complex: This relatively small group of patients (typically less than 5% of the population) requires the greatest attention. This group has multiple complex illnesses, and also suffer from psychosocial concerns or barriers. Patients in this population require intensive, pro-active care management.
2. High-risk: These patients have multiple risk factors that, if not managed, may result in transitioning into the highly complex group and typically describes about 20% of the population. This group can benefit from a structured care management program with one-on-one support to manage medical and social needs.
3. Rising risk: In this tier, patients may have one or several chronic conditions or risk factors and transition in and out of stability in their conditions.
4. Low risk: This group includes patients who are stable or healthy. The emphasis here is on keeping them healthy and engaged in the healthcare system without the use of unnecessary services.

There are multiple tools that can be used to assist in patient risk categorization:

- Hierarchical condition codes (HCC)
- Adjusted clinical groups (ACG)
- The Charlson Comorbidity Index
- The Chronic Comorbidity Count (CCC)

Patient-based artificial intelligence (AI) scoring is a relatively new development using AI as tool to predict patient outcomes.

Disease Management

Many illnesses lend themselves to proven protocols managed in consultation with physicians in specific specialties. Those protocols describe standard approaches to diagnosis and treatment, including the use of specific medications. Protocols can cover both outpatient and inpatient care. The protocols are typically adopted by physicians and used by their hospital medical staff, within their clinic, or both.

Utilization Management

Insurers have adopted utilization management techniques, such as prior authorization, to manage the cost of healthcare benefits by assessing care appropriateness before it is provided using evidence-based criteria or guidelines.

Utilization management staff typically work within a network of insurance plans, often referred to as a preferred network. The insurance company adopts clinician-developed, evidenced-based guidelines covering the appropriateness of specific diagnostic and treatment regimens, sometimes referred to as Medical Necessity Criteria, and they use that criteria to either authorize or deny care.

Plans to implement diagnostic tests and treatments noted above will require the physician to gain approval from the patient's insurance company. The insurance company compares the reasons that prompt the need for a diagnostic test, surgical intervention, or hospital admission with their adopted criteria. Based on that review, the insurance carrier will either approve or deny the procedure or admission.

Integrated Care Management

Integrated care management refers to the process of using care managers to coordinate the care of complex patients among a variety of settings and circumstances in order to deliver the right care in the right setting—which can result in reduced treatment costs.

In some cases, care managers are embedded in primary care practices to assist the other members of the care team in facilitating and coordinating the care of the patient. These primary care managers are typically funded through a per-member, per-month fee paid to a practice by insurance providers. On the hospital side, care managers, often in collaboration with those in the practice, coordinate patient needs post-discharge, which might include transfer to a lower acuity facility or home visits.

Leveraging Social Determinants of Health in Disease Management

While biological causes play a major role in patients' health, other factors contribute to the disease process and slow recovery after an illness or surgical procedure. These factors can include the patient's psychological condition and social/economic situation. Therefore, to achieve the best possible outcome for patients, physicians need to assess the psychosocial risk factors.

Clinicians can conduct a more complete patient assessment by implementing a health risk assessment or HRA. The HRA looks at a variety of factors to get a wholistic picture of the patient. Elements evaluated during an HRA include:

- Basic demographic characteristics
- Physical health
- Lifestyle behaviors
- Emotional health
- Social factors

When the clinician identifies patient gaps in emotional health or social factors, resources need to be identified to support the patient. Community benefit organizations (CBO) exist for this purpose. A CBO is a nonprofit charitable organization whose mission is solely to engage in community benefit activities. These can include relief agencies, places of worship, labor unions, teacher associations, community clubs, and veterans' groups.

Post-Acute Care Management

Given multiple imperatives to care for patients in the least acute and costly settings, healthcare executives can employ multiple strategies to facilitate care in the post-acute period:

- Home health: In some cases, patients need to augment what they and their family can do during recovery, such as change surgical dressings
- Heart failure clinics: Congestive heart failure patients require regular support and monitoring to avoid hospital readmissions
- Telehealth: There are a variety of solutions now available so that physicians can consult with patients and monitor patient parameters such as blood pressure or heart rate
- Skilled nursing facilities (SNF): In some cases, patients will need to go to a skilled nursing facility for the first stage of their recovery and then go home or to some other, less acute, setting
- Presurgical planning: For those patients whose surgery can be planned, the practice can arrange for post-op care prior to the procedure

Physicians can avail themselves of the hospital's discharge planning function to provide the right services.

Behavioral Health

According to a national survey conducted by McKinsey and Company, individuals who report poor mental health are more likely to use more health services, exhibiting significantly greater incidence of illness for hypertension, diabetes, and arthritis, and disproportionately using more healthcare resources.[11]

These patients benefit when there is trust in their care team, including timely and collaborative communication, stable housing and social support, and a focus on medication adherence. Recommendations for better managing patients in this population include:[12]

- Assign care managers
- Train PCPs in treating their unique needs
- Divert care away from the inpatient setting, as clinically appropriate
- Share actionable information in a timely manner, such as medication adherence
- Utilize community resources

Pharmacology, Lab Management, and Imaging

Appropriate utilization of medication, lab testing, and imaging can prove effective, not only in diagnosing and treating patients, but also in managing the cost of care.

Effective pharmaceutical management has been shown to reduce costs when there is active participation from pharmacists who have a both broad and deep understanding of therapeutic medication and disease management.[13] In addition, the use of generic medications can significantly reduce the cost of care.

Numerous brand medications in various therapeutic categories have generic therapeutic alternatives. However, with the rapidly changing environment, it is difficult for physicians to keep up to date with these offerings. Therefore, active pharmacist involvement can help.

Providers can look to two sources to determine the appropriateness of laboratory and imaging tests: accepted medical practice and payer requirements. Practices are best served when they take both sources into account, recognizing that the interests of accurate and timely diagnosis and treatment are of highest priority.

Disease-specific protocols as well as general preventive guidelines can be found in the medical literature or published by their medical societies and/or medical groups. At the same time, various payer policies may differ as to the appropriateness of different tests.

When providers are financially at risk for their prescribing decisions, if patients are under a capitation or other arrangement, the medical group should track cost and performance against other relevant metrics comparing the payer contract for each physician. These reports should occur no less often than quarterly and should be reviewed on a peer-to-peer basis.

Advanced Illness and Palliative Care

Advanced care planning and advance directives, which are patient initiated, provide guidance when the patient is unable to articulate their preferences due to incapacitation. Development of these directives also allows the patient to articulate their wishes to loved ones for their preferred level of care in the event of catastrophic illness and for end-of-life interventions. Advanced care planning defines the process for working through a plan with family and loved ones. Physicians should confirm that patients have these documents prepared, often with the help of an attorney. These directives should cover:

- The person to make care decisions when the patient can't
- The kind of medical treatment and intervention the patient wants or doesn't want
- How comfortable the patient wants to be
- How the patient wants people to treat them
- What the patient wants their loved ones to know

Hospice Care

Hospice care provides support to people in the final phase of a terminal illness, with a focus on comfort and quality of life. It is intended to meet the medical, emotional, social, practical, psychological, and spiritual needs of the patient and their family. Hospice care enables patients to be comfortable and free from pain, so that they live each day as fully as possible. Care can be provided in a hospice facility or at home.

Patients can be in hospice care for as long as six months. To be eligible for hospice, patients typically must meet specific criteria, sometimes depending on who is paying for the service.

Wellness and Prevention

Preventing illness in the first place creates a better quality of life for patients and families, and contributes to lower lifetime cost of care. Some health challenges faced by patients are genetic. Others are caused by learned habits or even a patient's socioeconomic position. Patients sometimes receive mixed messages through the media that encourage proper diet and exercise to enhance their health status. Physicians act as expert resources to help patients maintain a better quality of life.

Physicians may serve as the starting point in identifying health risks. Patients who need more time and detailed guidance can seek the support of a health coach and/or nutrition counselor.

Patient compliance can often hinge on how they perceive the care they receive. Practices can track patient reported outcomes (e.g., pain management, function, anxiety/depression) to determine the patient's quality of life following a procedure or other intervention.

Understanding the determinants of patient satisfaction can aid the clinician in tailoring care. When patients choose among treatment options, they may want to know the experiences and outcomes of other patients, for example.

Provider and Patient Engagement

The success of patient care strategies described in this section depend upon physician engagement. In their education and training, physicians learn the importance of weighing objective data as an aid to effective decision-making. Using data to manage care and measure success can cement physician engagement and commitment. Combining physician experience with timely and accurate reporting of patient-specific data will help improve care. At the same time, physicians need to have confidence in the accuracy and meaningfulness of the data.

A gap in care can be described as the difference between recommended best practices and the care that is provided. Examples include patients who skip seasonal vaccinations or age-related preventive screenings. Medical practices can measure these gaps using the Healthcare Effectiveness Data and Information Set (HEDIS), which is provided by the National Committee for Quality Assurance (NCQA). These metrics cover:

- Effectiveness of care
- Access/availability of care
- Experience of care
- Utilization and risk adjusted utilization
- Measures collected using electronic clinical data systems

Practices have implemented a variety of strategies to address gaps, including:

- Provider and patient reminders
- Provider and patient education
- Promotion of patient self-management
- Sharing data with providers, including regular audits and feedback
- Financial and regulatory incentives

Patient Engagement

Patients may be unaware of how to optimally utilize healthcare resources. Practices can assist and educate patients to assure them timely access and appropriate resources to help them better manage their health. In addition, many clinics now offer services that directly support patient engagement, including:

Extended Clinic Hours: In the past, medical clinics typically saw patients from 9 a.m. to 5 p.m. After hours care meant hospital emergency departments, which are a costlier, less effective option. Many practices now offer extended hours on certain weekdays, as well as offering hours on Saturday mornings. Typically, these clinics include only limited staff, depending on volume.

Digital connections: Many practices also offer telemedicine solutions to connect physicians with patients. Some practices have implemented "Call your Doctor First" campaigns to encourage checking in before going to the emergency department or urgent care center.

Annual Wellness Visits

Annual wellness visits provide a great opportunity for patients to get a regular checkup and discuss their health. These visits provide the clinician an opportunity to discuss concerns and conduct standard testing (e.g., bloodwork or other lab tests) to discover potential hidden problems, which can be addressed proactively and potentially decrease morbidity and costs while improving patient health.

Patient Education

Practices can engage patients in their own care through ongoing education efforts. Practices can share information that describes actions for patients to better manage their personal health through preventive care. Practices can also send targeted information to patients with specific chronic conditions (e.g., hypertension, obesity), as well as strategies to improve their condition. Practices can also engage with patients through the use of wearable health devices that track heart rate, blood pressure, and body temperature, as well as blood oxygen saturation, and physical activities.

Group Support

Some practices offer group support (sometimes referred to as cooperative healthcare clinics) for patients with certain chronic conditions, similar to group therapy, which psychiatrists and psychologists use. Patients can attend on a regular basis or some groups offer a "drop-in" option for patients to attend on an as-needed basis. In this setting, patients can learn from one another and can build self-management skills in discussion with their peers. In addition, many private insurers allow billing for group visits using the appropriate level of CPT code for an established office visit for each attendee.

SAMPLE QUESTIONS

1. **Model of care defines the way healthcare services are delivered. The basic principles of a model of care include:**

   A. Patient controlled

   B. Caregiver is centric

   C. Benefits system controlled

   D. Integrated care

2. **In an accountable care organization (ACO) network, who is ultimately responsible for the patient's care?**

   A. Physician team

   B. Patient

   C. Primary care physician

   D. Care coordinator

3. **In a patient-centered medical home (PCMH), treatment is coordinated through the:**

   A. Patient's family

   B. Hospital

   C. Insurance carrier

   D. Primary care physician

Answers: 1-D, 2-C, 3-D

TASK 2: PAYMENT MODELS

While fee-for-service reimbursement still dominates, a variety of modifications to that model have been adopted by a variety of payers over the past several years. Market pressures encourage improved processes and outcomes at lower price points. Insurers are creating payment models to provide incentives when the right care is delivered in the right location, at the right time and at the right cost.

This section explores various approaches to revise the method for paying physicians, with the intent to provide better incentives than in the traditional fee-for-service model. According to an American Medical Association policy brief based on its Physician Practice Benchmark Survey (2018), while 59% of physicians worked in practices receiving some revenue from an advanced payment model in 2016, an average of 71% of practice revenue reflected fee-for-service payments.[14] Joint contracting as a reimbursement strategy will be addressed in the Organizational Models section.

KEY TERMS

Bundled payments: A single negotiated payment for all services for a specified procedure or condition.

Capitation: A payment model in which a provider organization, or group of organizations, is paid a set amount for each enrolled person, per period of time, whether or not that person seeks care.

Fee-for-service: Traditional payment model that pays physicians and practices a set amount for each designated service or procedure.

Merit-based Incentive Payment Systems (MIPS): A Medicare program to provide incentives to practices that achieve performance standards and improvement.

Pay for performance (P4P): Insurers tie financial incentives or disincentives to performance as quantified against specific targets metrics.

Shared savings: Providers receive performance-based incentives to share cost savings and disincentives to share the excess costs of healthcare delivery.

Consider evaluating payment models using a matrix with increasing levels of accountability compared to increasing potential for risk and/or reward.

The fee-for-service model pays physicians based on a fee schedule tied to work output and CPT codes. In 2016, more than 80% of physicians worked in practices receiving at least some revenue from fee-for-service.[15]

Alternative payment models carry with them increasing levels of risk for physicians and their practices. These range from various pay for performance (P4P) approaches to capitation.

Figure 4.1

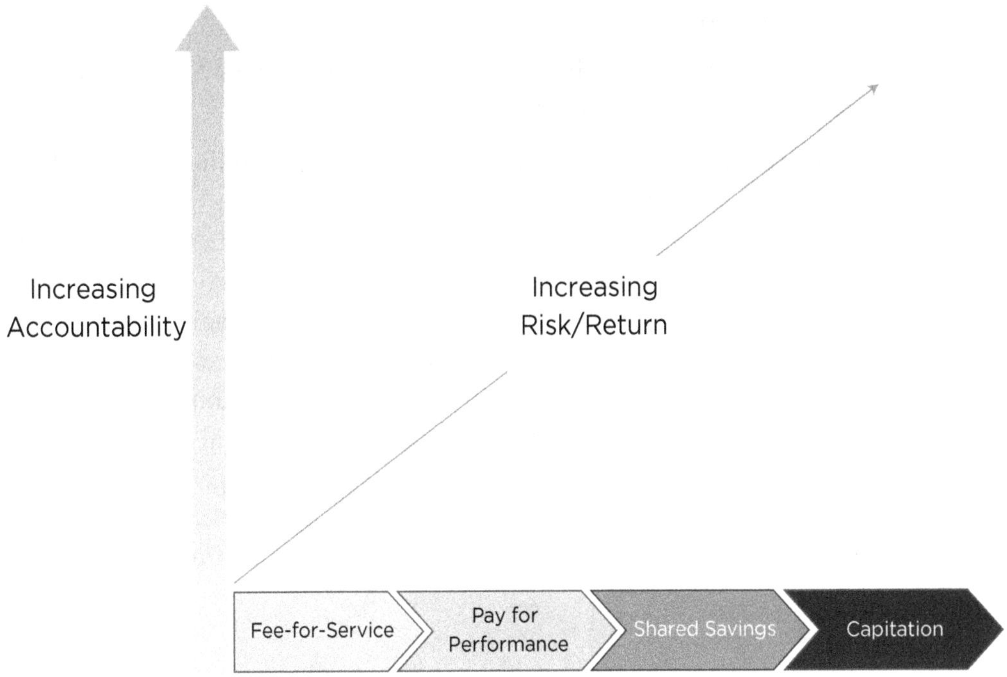

With increasing risk comes the requirement for advanced skills and capabilities along with the willingness to assume that risk. Physician groups need data to accurately track performance along with the capability to monitor and make changes when needed. In addition, they need the financial flexibility to weather risk, including the use of stop/loss insurance coverage. Practices would be well advised to learn from those who have taken on risk successfully.

Pay for Performance

Under pay-for-performance (P4P) approaches, insurers tie financial incentives or disincentives to performance, as quantified against specific targets. Under these arrangements, practices can earn adjustments to the fee-for-service rates, usually as bonuses. For example, Medicare utilizes two forms of P4P: Merit-based Incentive Payment System (MIPS) and Advanced Alternative Payment Models (APMs). Under MIPS, physicians are measured across four categories:

- Quality: Practice picks six measures of performance that best fit the practice based on performance measures created by CMS, as well as medical professional and stakeholder groups.
- Improvement activities: This includes activities that assess how the practice improves care processes, enhances patient engagement and increases access. Practices can choose the targets from categories such as enhancing care coordination, shared decision-making, and access expansion.

- Promoting interoperability: Focuses on patient engagement and the electronic exchange of health information using electronic health record technology.
- Cost: The cost of the care provided is calculated by CMS, based on the physician's Medicare claims.

In order to be included, physicians must meet eligibility criteria. Those criteria vary by clinician type and patient volume and must exceed low-volume thresholds.

Advanced alternative payment models (APMs) offer a 5% incentive and other APM-specific bonuses as well as exclusion from the MIPS reporting requirements and payment adjustment. If the practice achieves certain thresholds, they can become a Qualifying APM Participant (QP). Practices can qualify if they're certified as a Comprehensive Primary Care Plus organization, participate in a Medicare ACO, or the Medicare shared savings program, track 2, for example.[16]

Specialty groups can find P4P opportunities targeted for their specialty, whether primary care, medical, or surgical. For example, insurers can use value pathways to reward practices that adopt state of the art treatment protocols.

Shared Savings

Shared savings models can be described as the next-level of risk arrangements, under which providers receive performance-based incentives to share cost savings and disincentives to prevent excess costs of healthcare delivery.

Practices can also take advantage of shared savings opportunities, including one-sided contracts with upside only potential and two-sided contracts which also have downside risk but the potential for greater reward, as well. Often combined with fee-for-service, models such as P4P, bundled payments, global payments, or capitation, shared savings programs reward providers that reduce total healthcare expenditure on their patients below an expected level set by the payer.

The physician is then entitled to a share of the savings. The payer and physician agree on patient attribution, covered services, and projected medical costs. Claims are submitted as they would be under fee-for-service. The physician and payer review medical costs to see what, if any, savings were achieved. The insurer pays a bonus to all participants (e.g., primary care, specialists, and hospitals) based on savings achieved.

When a practice accepts downside risk, the agreed-upon budget requires the provider to cover a portion of costs if savings targets are not achieved. This portion could be either a percentage of the premium or a set amount. As expected, there is a relationship between risk and reward. Because under this model providers take on more risk, essentially upside and downside, most often the opportunity for upside financial gain is larger.

Shared savings programs, however, can suffer from several significant shortcomings:

- They may not pay for primary care services such as nurse care managers for chronic disease patients, and phone and email consults with other physicians.

- In many cases, they also require upfront spending by the provider to implement the processes or technologies necessary to achieve success.
- While revenue may increase from such programs, it could be months or years in the future before performance improvement has been assessed.
- Also, providers with the initially highest rates of hospital admissions, highest use of unnecessary procedures, and other wastes of resources benefit most under the shared-savings model. In contrast, the best performers (those with relatively low costs and high quality of care) have historically saved payers significant amounts of money but received no reward for doing so.

Bundled Payment

As its name suggests, the bundled payment, or episode of care model, provides a single negotiated payment for all services for a specified procedure or condition, such as pregnancy and birth, knee and hip replacement surgeries, and certain cardiac procedures. The model bases provider payment amounts on the costs of adhering to clinical standards of care, risk stratification, and complication allowances. It also incentivizes provider performance based on a comprehensive score card.

Under an episode-of-care payment system, physicians benefit from any savings they generate by improving efficiency within a specific episode of care. In some cases, they can also benefit from the savings they achieve by preventing unnecessary episodes of care. The payer, meanwhile, saves by paying the provider less per episode or per patient than it may have previously. As in the shared savings model, the practice may have to cover the costs of services for such procedures or conditions that exceed the agreed-upon reimbursement amount.

Capitation

Under capitation arrangements, a provider organization, or group of organizations, are paid a set amount for each enrolled person assigned to them, per period of time, whether or not that person seeks care. As a result, the providing organization takes on the full financial risk. Using actuarial analysis, a monthly fee is calculated (based on historical claims and acuity of the patient population) and paid to the organization. The organization then determines how to divide up the capitated payment. Like other models noted earlier, this disbursement is based on a combination of incentives and fee-for-service agreements.

There are two basic capitation models: global, or full capitation, and partial, or blended capitation. Regardless of whether the capitation is global or partial, the provider is at full risk for covered services.

- Under global capitation, the provider organization is paid a single fixed amount for all healthcare services a patient could receive including primary and specialty care, hospitalizations, and ancillary services.

- Under partial capitation, the monthly fee paid to the organization only covers a defined set of healthcare services. Services not covered are usually paid for on a fee-for-service basis. For example, it is not uncommon to see a partial capitation model that only includes physician services (primary care and specialty) and laboratory services, but excludes hospital-based care, pharmacy, and mental health benefits.

SAMPLE QUESTIONS

1. **What is the payment structure that shares risk between the payer and the provider?**

   A. Capitation

   B. Fee-for-service

   C. Bundled

   D. Deductible

2. **Providers are required to report in which category for the Merit-based Incentive Payment System (MIPS)?**

   A. Quality

   B. Relative value units (RVUs)

   C. Denials

   D. Charges

Answers: 1-C, 2-A

TASK 3: ORGANIZATIONAL MODELS

Market forces driven by both cost management and patient experience have led to innovative approaches to organizing care. The models described below can be considered approaches to organizing the delivery of patient care and how physician practices are owned, governed, and compensated. Practices should also consult with legal and tax professionals for advice to avoid or mitigate unanticipated risks.

KEY TERMS

Clinically integrated network (CIN): A mechanism that permits physicians and hospitals to contract jointly with payers to get better reimbursement rates if they meet specific qualification criteria.

Co-management (Co-M): Establish a means for physicians and hospitals to share management of a service line (e.g., cardiology, orthopedics) and the results of any improvement in performance.

Physician employment: Certain states permit the direct employment of physicians by health systems.

Designated health service: Clinical services specified under the Stark Law (such as clinical laboratory services, outpatient prescription drug services and physical and occupational therapy and imaging services). Physicians cannot refer patients to services payable by Medicare or Medicaid from entities with which the physician or an immediate family member has a financial relationship, unless an exception applies (e.g., in-office ancillary services).

Group practices: A legal arrangement between physicians who practice together.

Independent practice association (IPA): A legal entity owned by a network of independent physician practices, designed to reduce overhead and/or jointly pursue business ventures.

Management services organization (MSO): Provides administrative services to physician practices, such as financial management, revenue cycle management, and human resources support.

Professional service agreement (PSA): In states that don't permit physician employment by health systems, physicians can join a PSA and receive many of the same benefits as employment.

Group Practices

For physicians to participate in a group practice, they need to satisfy certain legal requirements. As a group practice, physicians can contract as a group with payers and thus negotiate better rates than they might on their own. Section

411.352 of the Federal Code specifies that a group practice must meet certain conditions:

- The group practice must consist of a single legal entity operating primarily for the purpose of being a physician group practice in any organizational form (e.g., corporate, partnership). The legal form the practice chooses must be recognized by the state in which the group practice achieves its legal status.
- The group practice must have at least two physicians who are members of the group. Each physician must provide the full range of patient care services through the joint use of shared office space, facilities, equipment, and personnel. Services must be billed under a billing number assigned to the group, and the amounts received must be treated as receipts of the group.
- Patient care services must be measured by one of the following:
    - The total time each member spends on patient care services
    - Any reasonable alternative measure, which must be determined in advance, applied consistently over time, verifiable, and documented
- The overhead expenses of and income from the practice must be distributed according to methods determined before the receipt of payment for the services.
- The group practice must be a unified business with centralized decision-making by a body representative of the group practice that maintains effective control over the group's assets and liabilities (including, but not limited to, budgets, compensation, and salaries) and consolidated billing, accounting, and financial reporting.
- Physicians cannot receive compensation directly or indirectly based on the volume or value of their referrals. They can be paid productivity bonuses and profit shares. A physician in the group practice may be paid a share of overall profits of the group, provided that the share is not determined in any manner that is directly related to the volume or value of referrals of designated health service. A physician in the group practice may be paid a productivity bonus based on services that they have personally performed. The group should consult legal counsel to assure compliance with the various nuances of this requirement.

Independent Practice Association

An independent physician association (IPA) is a legal entity owned by a network of independent physician practices. It is designed to reduce overhead and/or jointly pursue business ventures such as contracts with employers, accountable care organizations (ACO), and/or managed care organizations (MCOs).

An IPA allows physicians who aren't part of a corporate entity to enjoy some of the same benefits as a larger organization. IPAs allow physicians to practice independently, take on payer contracts they might not be able to service on their own, and potentially reduce overhead. Payers are more likely to sign contracts with larger groups of physicians who can provide comprehensive services, demonstrate high quality outcomes, assume risk, and provide unique, innovative, or collaborative healthcare services.

IPAs must be of significant size and be able to demonstrate effective care management that results in reduced medical expenses in order to appeal to payers.

Management Service Organizations

Management service organizations (MSO) are created to provide administrative services to physician practices. MSOs can benefit practices by:

1. Focusing leadership's attention on day-to-day office operations and avoiding the challenge of frequent administrative distractions
2. Using economies of scale and expertise, MSOs can offer more effective services at a lower cost

Common MSO offerings can include:

- Financial management
- Human resources and personnel management
- Staff education and training
- Revenue cycle
- Regulatory compliance
- Managed care contracting including credentialing and contract management
- Group purchasing
- Risk management

When considering joining an MSO, healthcare executives should consider the advantages, disadvantages, and requirements to manage the outsourced services, as well as the cost.[17]

Potential Advantages:

- Expertise in the services to be purchased
- Ability to focus management's time on other matters
- Improved revenue/cost profile

Potential Disadvantages:

- Temporary performance improvement and/or non-performance requiring revisiting the decision
- Criticism from practice owners due to non-performance or adjustment to inevitable changes

Additional Considerations:

- Establish a well-defined scope

- Define disciplined accountability
- Clarify the cost
- Document in the contract
- Conduct due diligence
- Involve physicians

Co-Management

Co-management (Co-M) arrangements establish a means for physicians and hospitals to share governance of a service line (e.g., cardiology, orthopedics) and the results of any improvement in performance. Under this arrangement, physicians actively participate in decision-making and can benefit financially from success in service line initiatives. Co-M arrangements can be housed in a separate entity, or a hospital can use professional service agreements (PSAs).

Under a Co-M arrangement:

- Physicians retain their practice assets, structure, governance, and compensation structure
- Private practice and employed physicians can participate
- Membership/ownership can be by individual physician or by group
- Physicians can continue to practice at other hospitals
- Physicians have a greater role in service line direction, though ultimate authority still rests with the health system board
- Physicians elect physician representatives to lead and develop guidelines; there is less individual autonomy than in private practice

These arrangements focus on improving clinical performance, reducing cost, and enhancing patient satisfaction. Co-management provides oversight for a particular service line. For example, a cardiac services Co-M might oversee the cardiac catheterization lab, cardiac surgical operations, diagnostic testing, inpatient care, and cardiac disease management.

Physicians, working with hospital staff, develop initiatives to improve performance. Recognizing that commitment of time and effort comes at a cost, physicians have the opportunity to be paid for their efforts (within fair market value constraints) for both their commitment of time and achievement of goals covering improvements in performance. In addition to hourly pay for physician time, hospitals often use a pool of dollars to compensate participating physicians for achievement of jointly developed and pre-set targets covering clinical, financial, and patient experience metrics.

The collaborative nature of Co-M positions allows physicians to benefit under at-risk contracting and to have a greater say in how their hospital organizes operations and serves their patients.

Figure 4.2

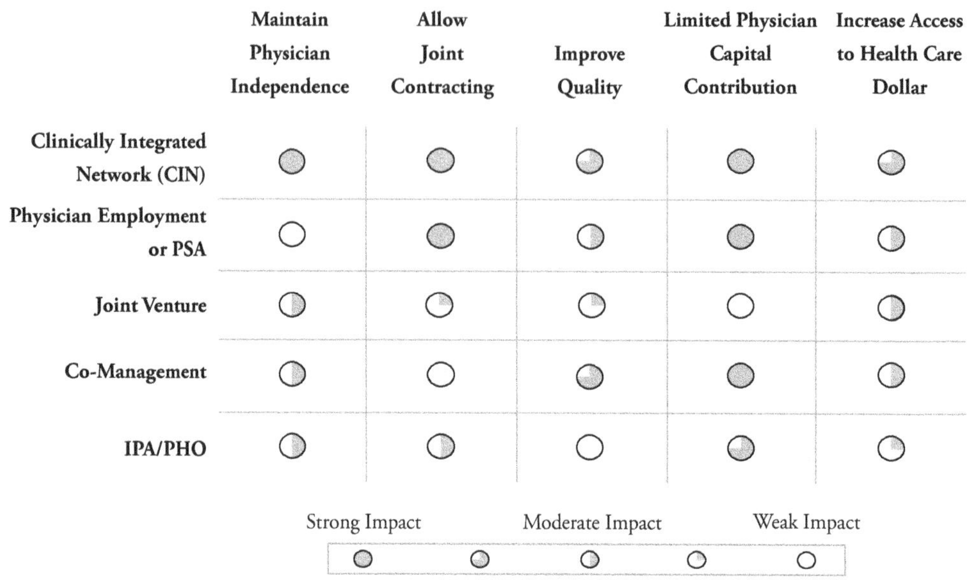

Clinically Integrated Networks

Clinically integrated networks (CINs) allow physicians and hospitals to contract jointly with payers to get better reimbursement rates, but only if they meet certain criteria established by the Federal Trade Commission (FTC). More specifically, a CIN is a population health management and contracting entity that connects a set of providers across the entire care continuum through information, clinical standards and protocols, and care management services to help patients navigate health services, while simultaneously improving cost, quality, and outcomes (the Triple Aim) for the communities and populations served by the network.

CINs allow physician and hospital providers to retain their independent organizations yet jointly demonstrate value, contract, and offer new health plan options for payers, employers, and individuals seeking value-based care.

In order to qualify as a CIN, the Federal Trade Commission requires an entity to:

- Demonstrate an active and ongoing program to evaluate and modify practice patterns by the network's physician participants and create a high degree of interdependence and cooperation among the physicians to control costs and ensure quality
- This program may include:
  - Establishing mechanisms to monitor and control utilization of healthcare services that are designed to control costs and assure quality of care
  - Choosing network physicians who are likely to further these efficiency objectives
  - Invest capital, both monetary and human, in the necessary infrastructure and capability to realize the claimed efficiencies

CINs serve their in-network providers in four primary functional areas:

- Network development: Building a network of healthcare providers across all specialties and sites of care to provide increased access for patients
- Information and performance management: Integrating and analyzing healthcare information from all network providers to reduce duplication of services and track and improve the cost, quality, and health of the populations served
- Care management: Integrating clinical processes, protocols, and services to coordinate patient care effectively and efficiently
- Financial and risk management: Financial and actuarial management services to develop, execute, and manage health insurance products/ contracts

Supplemental to these functional areas are four key principles of every CIN:

- Provider responsibilities: Active participation, engagement, and time committed to enhancing clinical quality (care pathways) and reducing costs
- Provider accountability: CIN standards of participation create recourse if providers are noncompliant in quality and cost reduction policies defined by the CIN
- Clinical quality standardization: The organization must demonstrate that the CIN improves quality and efficiency over time
- Resource use: The organization must make efforts to meet quality standardization and cost efficiencies, including infrastructure investment, efficient network participants, and clinical improvement

A clinically integrated network is not:

- A merger or acquisition of existing provider assets
- A physician employment mechanism.
- A physician practice management company
- An exclusive arrangement

Health System Employment/Professional Services Agreement

According to one survey, physicians typically seek hospital employment for the following reasons:[18]

1. The overhead and cost of maintaining a medical practice was too high (33%)
2. They wanted to focus on the practice of medicine and patient care, rather than administrative hassles (27%)
3. There were too many reimbursement cuts (26%)

Under an employment or a professional services agreement (PSA), physicians no longer own their practice. Instead, a health system or PSA controlled by a health system employs them. PSAs employ physicians in states where the Medical Practice Act does not allow the corporate practice of medicine (e.g., California and Texas).

Whether employed by a health system or under a PSA, physicians function as employees similar to any other staff positions. Executives (who may or may not be licensed physicians) make decisions under direction from a board of directors governing work schedules, services offered, compensation, and employment and supervision of practice staff.

To avoid the appearance of paying physicians for referrals, the federal government enacted laws (known as the Stark provisions or Stark Law). Under employment arrangements, physicians can only be paid at a rate determined to be "fair market value" and "commercially reasonable." Please see a more detailed description concerning the Stark regulations in the *Risk and Compliance Management* volume of the Body of Knowledge Review Series.

SAMPLE QUESTIONS

1. **The most accurate definition of a clinically integrated network is:**

   A. A group of providers whose goal is to demonstrate high quality and efficiency

   B. A subset of a larger provider group

   C. A network of providers working together with the common goal of improving the health of a specific population

   D. A network created by and for a specific employer/client group

2. **Clinical integration is "the means to facilitate the coordination of patient care across conditions, providers, settings, and time in order to achieve care that is safe, timely, effective, efficient, equitable, and patient-focused." A key component to the success of clinical integration is:**

   A. The location of the practice

   B. Data integration

   C. The ratio of physicians to support staff

   D. Whether the practice is part of a large healthcare network or is independent

Answers: 1-A, 2-B

TASK 4: INNOVATION AND EMERGING TECHNOLOGIES

Both the healthcare system, in general, and medical groups, in particular, can benefit from and will also be challenged by rapid advances in clinical and information technology. Consumer/patient demand for increased connection and information will drive nontraditional approaches for the delivery of care. This section highlights many of these trends.

Note: Given the rapidity of innovation and the uncertainty of what lies ahead, this section could become dated quickly. The successful healthcare executive must stay abreast of these rapidly evolving developments. Professional societies are often a great way to learn of the latest developments.

KEY TERMS

Artificial intelligence (AI): The use of computer based, complex algorithms to diagnose and treat patients.

Blockchain: A distributed digital ledger system where blocks of information contain transactions that can be securely shared between parties.

Quantum computing: Enables computers to utilize broader sets of data at much faster speeds, based on the fundamental principles of quantum physics.

Telemedicine: Use of telecommunication technology and remote access for consultation, diagnosis, and treatment of patients by medical professionals.

3D printing: Computer-based printing technology that utilizes various materials to physically craft customizable items. Medical uses include orthopedics support and, potentially, organs and pharmaceuticals.

Telemedicine/Telehealth

Care that has traditionally been provided in the physician's office is now moving closer to consumers. The Centers for Medicare and Medicaid Services (CMS) considers telehealth (or telemonitoring) as the use of information and telecommunication technology for remote access to diagnosis, consultation, and treatment, including remote patient monitoring. In fact, practices can now bill for telemedicine visits including the same basis as face-to-face interactions.

Telemedicine differs from the more general concept of telehealth. The American Telemedicine Association defines telemedicine as "the use of medical information exchanged from one site to another via electronic communications to improve patients' health status."[19]

One might also hear the term "telehealth," which covers a broader definition of remote healthcare and may not involve clinical services. Video conferencing;

transmission of still images; e-health, including patient portals; remote monitoring of vital signs; continuing medical education; and nursing call centers are all considered part of telemedicine and telehealth.[20]

Telemedicine has the potential to benefit traditionally difficult to reach communities, such as rural, homebound, and underserved populations, though access to the internet and video technology can present a barrier.

Mobile Units

Mobile units provide another solution to the lack of access. A mobile health clinic can be defined as a doctor's office located inside a large van, bus, or RV. These vehicle-based clinics can be independent or sponsored by health systems.

A review of the literature[21] supports the efficacy of these clinics. As a result of increasing access, these programs have seen patient improvements in preventative care and the management of chronic disease.

Data Aggregation from Disparate EMR Sources

Electronic medical records operate on a variety of hardware and software platforms. At the same time, coordinating patient care among a variety of physicians and other institutions requires the accurate and timely exchange of data.

Fast Healthcare Interoperability Resources (FHIR) provides the standard for exchanging healthcare information electronically as the latest framework being adopted by the healthcare community to advance interoperability.[22] FHIR offers several benefits:

- Providers can achieve real-time access to quality data.
- Practices can realize some relief from the burden of reporting quality measures. FHIR aligns CMS Electronic Clinical Quality Measurement (eCQM) reporting with the standard industry clinical data exchange framework, and it enables automated data retrieval from EHRs along with submissions of quality data, through use of standards-based application programming interfaces (APIs).

Artificial Intelligence

Artificial intelligence (AI) is playing a growing role in the delivery of patient care, taking on simple tasks and aiding in more complicated decision-making. This list captures some of the potential ways in which AI may impact the industry:

- Predictive modeling and patient risk stratification:[23] Uses both clinical and financial data to better predict utilization and costs of healthcare for certain kinds of patients.
- Robot-Assisted Surgery: Robotic surgery, or robot-assisted surgery, enables doctors to perform many types of complex procedures with greater precision and control than is possible with conventional techniques.[24]

- Virtual Nursing Assistants: An AI-powered virtual nursing assistant helps to identify illness based on symptoms, monitors health status, conducts virtual wellness checks, and schedules physician appointments. In addition, the patient can ask the virtual nursing assistant to guide them through a process to better understand what they are going through.[25]
- Administrative Workflow Assistance: Through automation of administrative workflow, providers can prioritize urgent matters and save time on routine tasks such as voice-to-text.[26]
- Dosage error reduction: AI augments clinical decision-making around prescriptions.
- Connected machines: Patients benefit from connecting AI platforms to medical devices, such as critical care and wearable devices, to more closely monitor their conditions and alert caregivers to the need for intervention.
- Preliminary diagnosis: In addition to AI advances in medical imaging, these systems possess a wealth of data from patients and the medical literature, and can process the information far faster and more effectively than medical professionals.[27] Innovations include the use of radiology or pathology images (microscope images) to accurately diagnose patient conditions such as in oncology.
- Automated image diagnosis: As of this writing, it's estimated approximately one-third of hospitals and imaging centers use AI in the diagnosis process.[28] Radiologists use AI technologies to sift through images for potential abnormalities and patterns, increasing diagnostic accuracy and saving time.

Sensors and Wearable Technology

Wearable devices provide real time monitoring of health parameters. In addition to fitness trackers, wearable devices can include monitors that track cardiac rhythm, blood pressure, temperature, respiration rates, and glucose for diabetic patients. Patients with sleep apnea use continuous positive airway pressure (CPAP) machines. These devices can transmit information to providers continuously (e.g., glucose monitoring) or periodically (e.g., CPAP).

Physicians often struggle to help patients change their health behaviors, whether it be to quit smoking, lose weight, or exercise more. But combining behavioral economics and "gamification" — putting game elements such as points and achievement levels into non-game contexts — holds promise for driving behavior change when a doctor's advice, and patient's good intentions, are not enough.[29] This approach uses gaming techniques from other industries to encourage behaviors and social elements to reinforce behaviors.

Remote Monitoring Tools

Remote patient monitoring (RPM) uses technology to monitor patient health outside of the traditional clinical setting. Common examples of remote patient monitoring devices include voice apps that remind diabetes patients to take their insulin while allowing their physician to monitor the disease and digital blood pressure cuffs that enable patients to remotely send physicians their blood pressure and pulse measurements.

3D Printing

3D printing involves programming a computer to apply multiple layers of a specific material (often plastic or metal powders), molding them one layer at a time into a final product. Medical solutions include:

- Customized prosthetics: Prosthetics can now be tailored to a patient's unique body measurements for better fit and greater comfort.
- Bioprinting and tissue engineering: Medical research is now harnessing this technology to build tiny organs, or "organoids," using stem cells as the production material. Researchers expect that one day, these organoids, will grow inside the body of patient and take over when an organ, such as a kidney or liver, fails. Researchers, working with a biological ink that contains both human plasma and material extracts taken from skin biopsies, were able to print about 100 square centimeters of human skin which could benefit burn victims.
- Pharmaceutical printing: Often, patients take multiple medications to treat multiple ailments and need to take the medications at different times of the day to avoid drug interactions. A 3D-printed pill, unlike a traditionally manufactured capsule, may, one day, contain multiple drugs, each with different release times. This so-called "polypill" concept has already been tested for patients with diabetes and is showing promise.

Though this may read like science fiction, these interventions show great promise.[30]

Quantum Computing

Quantum computing can exponentially advance computational power and promises to usher in a new age in computing technology.[31] It is a revolutionary concept in digital data processing based on the fundamental principles of quantum physics, enabling computers to utilize broader sets of data at much faster speeds.

The benefits for healthcare include:

- Supporting medical imaging, with the ability to tap into more data from digital images such as MRI and CT
- Sequencing and analyzing DNA
- Accelerating drug design through review of multiple clinical trials and corresponding DNA data
- Using predictive analytics in which reams of data can be analyzed quickly to arrive at more accurate diagnosis and treatment approaches

Blockchain

In simplest terms, blockchain is a distributed digital ledger system where transactions between parties of various types exchange information and are recorded redundantly in multiple databases that are slow but secure.[32] It provides a reliable and safe means for multiple parties to review data. Potential benefits in healthcare include:

- Greater security for patient data in support of HIPAA restrictions
- Enhanced collaboration and quality of information among providers in different locations

Using interoperability standards, smart contracts, and cryptographic identities, patients can securely exchange data with providers and regulate access. The resulting comprehensive, longitudinal medical records can significantly improve the cost and quality of patient care for individuals and populations alike.[33] Blockchain also provides the opportunity for patients to both own and control the content in their medical record, with comprehensive access to their profiles and history.

SAMPLE QUESTIONS

1. The use of telemedicine within the healthcare delivery system is experiencing unprecedented growth. Telemedicine technology includes all of the following except:

A. Simple telephone calls

B. Mailed letters

C. Video conferencing equipment

D. Secure, high-tech apps

2. The primary aim of health-related artificial intelligence applications is to analyze relationships between:

A. Diagnosis and treatment

B. Treatment techniques and patient outcomes

C. Software and hardware

D. Physicians and patients

Answers: 1-B, 2-B

TRANSFORMATIVE HEALTHCARE DELIVERY QUIZ

1. The term "social determinants of health" is most effectively defined as:

A. The number of healthy friends a person has

B. Social and economic factors that influence a person's health status

C. A person's eating habits when in a social setting

D. The level of a person's involvement in community activities and how it determines their health status

2. What are the three core elements that the triple aim focuses on improving?

A. Patient experience, health of populations, cost of care

B. Insurance reimbursement, patient experience, employee health

C. Patient experience, cost of care, employee experience

D. Staffing metrics, physician satisfaction, employee experience

3. Which is an example of an advanced payment model (APM)?

A. Fee-for-service

B. Medicare reimbursement

C. Accountable care organization

D. Private pay model

4. An example of an insurance contracting model is:

A. Bundled payments

B. Medicare fee schedule

C. Accountable care organization

D. Affordable Care Act

ANSWERS

1-B: Genetics are responsible for some health conditions; however, even genetics can be impacted by social determinants. For example, there is clear evidence that those with more limited access to healthcare (e.g., those without insurance) suffer worse outcomes.

2-A: The goal of the Triple AIM is to simultaneously improve cost, quality, and outcomes for the communities and populations served by the network.

3-C: The other three options reflect more traditional forms of payment for services. An accountable care organization typically will reimburse for metrics not only related to cost and work effort, but for "value," such as quality or avoiding hospitalization.

4-A: Bundled payments refer to a single, comprehensive payment for one episode of care. None of the others is a model, though each may include bundled payments as one method of reimbursement.

Notes

1. "Accountable Care Organizations (ACOs): General Information," The Centers for Medicare & Medicaid Services, https://innovation.cms.gov/innovation-models/aco.
2. "Overview Shared Savings Program,"; The Centers for Medicare & Medicaid Services, https://www.cms.gov/Medicare/Medicare-Fee-for-Service-Payment/sharedsavingsprogram/index?redirect=/sharedsavingsprogram.
3. Higgins T, Schottenfeld and L., Crosson J., "Primary Care Practice Facilitation Curriculum Module 25: The Patient-Centered Medical Home: Principles and Recognition Processes," September 2015, https://pcmh.ahrq.gov/page/defining-pcmh, https://pcmh.ahrq.gov/sites/default/files/attachments/pcpf-module-25-pcmh-principles.pdf.
4. "Key functions of a Medical Home – Access and Continuity," American Academy of Family Practice, https://www.aafp.org/practice-management/transformation/pcmh/key-functions/access-continuity.html.
5. Smith C., Balatbat C., Corbridge S., Dopp A., Fried J., Harter R., Landefeld S., Martin C., Opelka F., Sandy L., Sato L. and Sinsky C., "Implementing Optimal Team-Based Care to Reduce Clinician Burnout," National Academy of Medicine, September 17, 2018, https://nam.edu/implementing-optimal-team-based-care-to-reduce-clinician-burnout.
6. "How to Use Team-Based Care to Improve the Patient Experience," Patient Engagement HIT – Xtelligent Health Care Media, https://patientengagementhit.com/news/how-to-use-team-based-care-to-improve-the-patient-experience.
7. "Planned Care and Population Health," American Academy of Family Practice, https://www.aafp.org/practice-management/transformation/pcmh/key-functions/planned-care-population-health.html.
8. Meyers D., Peikes D., Genevro J., Peterson G., Taylor E., Lake T., Smith K. and Grumbach K., "The Roles of Patient-Centered Medical Homes and Accountable Care Organizations in Coordinating Patient Care," Agency for Healthcare Research and Quality, December 2010, https://pcmh.ahrq.gov/sites/default/files/attachments/Roles%20of%20PCMHs%20And%20ACOs%20in%20Coordinating%20Patient%20Care.pdf.
9. Kindig D. and Stoddart G, "What is population health?" American Journal of Public Health, March 2003, 93 (3): 380-3.

10. "Population Health Risk Stratification Guide," National Association of Community Health Centers, http://www.nachc.org/wp-content/uploads/2019/03/Risk-Stratification-Action-Guide-Mar-2019.pdf.
11. Jones A., MD, "Insights on Mental Health from a 2019 McKinsey Consumer Survey," Presentation to the Medical Home Network, 2019.
12. Ibid.
13. Dalton K. and Byrne S., "Role of the Pharmacist in Reducing Healthcare Costs: Current Insights," Integrated Pharmacy Research and Practice, 2017, 6: 37-46, published online Jan. 25, 2017, https://www.ncbi.nlm.nih.gov/pmc/articles/PMC5774321.
14. "2018 Benchmark Survey," American Medical Association, https://www.ama-assn.org/about/research/physician-practice-benchmark-survey.
15. Ibid.
16. "Advanced Alternative Payment Models (APMs), Centers for Medicare & Medicaid Services, https://qpp.cms.gov/apms/advanced-apms.
17. "Understanding Management Services Organizations (MSOs)," Physicians Practice, April 27, 2016, https://www.physicianspractice.com/understanding-management-services-organizations-msos.
18. Manoj J., "Doctors in Private Practices are Now Joining Hospital Staffs," The Washington Post, March 12, 2012, https://www.washingtonpost.com/national/health-science/doctors-in-private-practices-are-now-joining-hospital-staffs/2012/02/14/gIQAEFz074_story.html.
19. Majorowicz A. and Tracy S., "Telemedicine: Bridging Gaps in Healthcare Delivery," American Health Information Management Association, http://library.ahima.org/doc?oid=100028#.Xp3Pr8hKi70.
20. Ibid.
21. Yu S., Hill C., Ricks M., Bennet J. and Oriol N., "The Scope and Impact of Mobile Health Clinics in the United States: A Literature Review, International Journal of Equity Health, 2017, vol.16:178, https://www.ncbi.nlm.nih.gov/pmc/articles/PMC5629787.
22. "Fast Healthcare Interoperability Resources (FHIR)," ECQI Resource Center, Centers for Medicare & Medicaid Services, https://ecqi.healthit.gov/fhir.
23. Kent J., "Deep Learning Bests Traditional Models in Risk Stratification," Health IT Analytics: Xtelligent Health Care Media, https://healthitanalytics.com/news/deep-learning-bests-traditional-models-in-risk-stratification; Chen J. and Asch S., "Machine Learning and Prediction in Medicine – Beyond the Peak of Inflated Expectations," New England Journal of Medicine: June 29, 2017, 376(26): 2507-2509, https://www.ncbi.nlm.nih.gov/pmc/articles/PMC5953825.
24. "Robotic Surgery," Mayo Clinic, https://www.mayoclinic.org/tests-procedures/robotic-surgery/about/pac-20394974.
25. "How AI-Powered Virtual Assistants Can Transform Healthcare," Avnet, February 2019, https://www.avnet.com/wps/portal/apac/resources/article/how-ai-powered-virtual-assisants-can-transform-healthcare.
26. "The Three Most Valuable Applications of AI in Healthcare," VentureBeat, https://venturebeat.com/2018/04/22/the-3-most-valuable-applications-of-ai-in-health-care.
27. Karkovnya O., "Artificial Intelligence & Deep Learning for Medical Diagnosis," 2019, https://towardsdatascience.com/artificial-intelligence-deep-learning-for-medical-diagnosis-9561f7a4e5f.
28. "One-third of Organizations use Artificial Intelligence in Medical Imaging," Health IT Analytics: Xtelligent Health Care Media, https://healthitanalytics.com/news/one-third-of-orgs-use-artificial-intelligence-in-medical-imaging.
29. Patel M., Chang S. and Volpp K., "Improving Healthcare by Gamifying It," *Harvard Business Review*, 2019, https://hbr.org/2019/05/improving-health-care-by-gamifying-it.
30. "How 3D Printing is Revolutionizing Healthcare as we Know It," TechCrunch, 2018, https://techcrunch.com/2018/04/05/bioprinted-organs-skin-and-drugs-how-3d-printing-is-revolutionizing-healthcare-as-we-know-it.
31. Solenov D., Breiler J. and Scherer J., "The Potential of Quantum Computing and Machine learning to Advance Clinical Research and Change the Practice of Medicine," Missouri Medicine, 2018 Sep-Oct, 115(5): 463-467, https://www.ncbi.nlm.nih.gov/pmc/articles/PMC6205278.
32. "Explain Blockchain in Simple English," Cryptosoftwares, https://www.quora.com/What-is-blockchain-in-very-simple-terms.
33. Hylok R. and Zeng X., "A Blockchain Framework for Patient-Centered Health Records and Exchange (HealthChain): Evaluation and Proof-of-Concept Study," Journal of Medical Internet Research, Volume 21, No. 8, 2019 (August), https://www.jmir.org/2019/8/e13592.

Chapter 5

Risk and Compliance Management

Risk and compliance management is not a new concept in medical practices. However, there's much uncertainty about the depth, breadth, and scope of work needed to maintain an effective compliance program. And while many of the same regulations and skills are required for managers in any organization, there are particular nuances specific to the delivery of healthcare in a clinic setting that differentiate healthcare executives from their peers in other business or healthcare delivery environments.

This section provides a blueprint designed by practicing healthcare executives to describe the key competencies, knowledge, and skills required to develop and maintain effective operations in the medical practice.

The major areas of competence in risk and compliance management, as identified by the certified and Fellowed members of the Medical Group Management Association (MGMA), are:

1. Facilitate the Corporate Legal Structure and the Governance for the Organization
2. Compliance with Applicable Laws and Regulations
3. Accreditation, Credentialing, and Licensing (Individuals and Organizations)
4. Emergency Preparedness
5. Cybersecurity

TASK 1: FACILITATE THE CORPORATE LEGAL STRUCTURE AND THE GOVERNANCE FOR THE ORGANIZATION

Healthcare executives should understand that all employees of the practice are responsible for doing their part to minimize risk and comply with applicable laws and regulations. Therefore, healthcare executives should try to create a culture in which all employees are open to risk management and compliance by encouraging open communication among and between all employees. Employees should be able to mention potential issues without fear of retaliation or other repercussions. This environment starts with the healthcare executive and spreads throughout the practice.

Practices must also designate people who are responsible for monitoring, updating, and communicating the risk and compliance plans for the organization. To comply with HIPAA regulations, for example, the practice must have a designated person who is in charge of maintaining the practice's compliance with HIPAA requirements. When it comes to safety, the practice should have one or more persons who perform the same tasks related to safety. Designating these individuals is an important part of the risk implementation and maintenance plan.

KEY TERMS

Application service provider (ASP): Vendor that provides applications and services via the internet.

Disaster: An event that prevents normal functioning.

1.1 Risk Management Program Implementation and Maintenance

To fully appreciate the ramifications and breadth of issues involved in risk management, it is essential to understand the four essential components of the risk management process:

1. Risk assessment and analysis: The identification and analysis of exposures
2. Loss control: A risk management technique that seeks to reduce the possibility that a loss will occur and reduce the severity of those that do occur
3. Risk financing: Using selected techniques, including financing, for failed control of losses
4. Monitoring: The continuous observation of selected methods for controlling losses for potential improvement[1]

These components, applied to financial, human, operational, technological, and strategic areas and property across all aspects of the organization, create the constellation that defines the organization's risk management program. They are all related to the healthcare executive's ability to assess risks.

On a scale smaller but more relevant to all practices are the preventable failures that result in medication errors, staff member injury, failure of service initiatives, or loss of business productivity as the result of technology failures. In each of those circumstances, the blame is often laid on the person who "didn't follow the policy" or "didn't pay close enough attention." In fact, processes without risk control mechanisms to counter the human factor are fraught with latent errors.

The opportunities for errors are frequently coincidental occurrences or arise through a series of small human errors that can ultimately result in devastating outcomes and losses. Reason's Swiss cheese model, often quoted in patient safety literature, is applicable to all aspects of an organization's processes and activities. The alignment of any number of process holes can result in risk management exposures. The key is to find and correct those exposures before losses occur.[2]

The most exhaustive way to identify potential exposures in complex systems is through a process, such as a Failure Modes and Effects Analysis (FMEA). This process, which gained popularity through its use in engineering, is designed to examine every step of a process and identify the myriad ways in which each step could fail, as well as the potential for that failure to be stopped.[3]

Unfortunately, use of process tools such as FMEA is limited by resources. Such analyses take time. Information on exposures that have high loss potential can be gathered from a number of sources. The organization's insurance claims and malpractice loss reports are basic sources of information. Complaints from patients and/or staff members are another fundamental source of information. Formal risk assessments by outside consultants, self-assessment questionnaires, literature reviews, and insurance application forms also provide exposure identification. Furthermore, by examining the questions on the insurance application or survey forms, the healthcare executive can ascertain which processes are perceived as high risk by insurers and other surveyors. Finally, by using a simple but effective technique, staff members can list the various processes in each department and then ask, "What can go wrong?" for each process.

The next step in the risk management process is to analyze the data and identify the tools that will reduce the frequency (loss prevention)[4] or the severity (loss reduction)[5] of losses. The potential losses that benefit most from these techniques are:

(1) Events that occur frequently but the cost per loss may be small (e.g., missed appointments or unplanned employee absences)

(2) Events that occur infrequently but are costlier per loss (e.g., medical malpractice claims or equipment failures)

Furthermore, any process with complex procedures or a complex environment that relies heavily on human compliance is subject to great variability and potential error.

The key point to remember is that loss control methods are not uniformly applicable in all situations. The unique location, culture, and characteristics of each organization may render a solution a potentially bad fit. Consequently, each solution must be analyzed for its potential latent failures in the given situation.

Most healthcare executives are familiar with the opportunities to finance risk through commercial insurance and self-insured vehicles, such as captives, risk retention groups, and trusts. What many healthcare executives may not fully appreciate, however, is that commercial insurance, although costlier, is effectively a contractual transfer of risk.[6] The risk of loss belongs to the insurer. Consequently, the risk of financial devastation through catastrophic events is minimized for the organization.

The downside to risk transfer is that the insurance company maintains control over what will be covered and retains the ability to increase premiums. Furthermore, the premium paid by the organization is not based solely on the organization's history, nor specifically on its loss control efforts, but on an aggregate of similar organizations with combined loss experience.

For forms of losses that are unpredictable and potentially costly (e.g., automobiles, directors' and officers' liability, employment liability, property, key person), commercial insurance is the standard and probably the most cost-effective form of financing risk. The organization hopes to never need it. Nonetheless, it would be extremely difficult to predict ultimate losses and to plan for setting aside sufficient funds to cover these losses should they occur.

Self-insurance vehicles are best when there is a known frequency and consistent value of typical losses.[7] The organization must have sufficient funds or reserve set aside to cover those losses.

In addition, there are losses that occur infrequently but result in such large costs that it is better to cover them with more structured forms of risk financing. For minimal losses or extremely infrequent losses, risk financing might include loans, nonfunded reserves, or even payment from the operations budget.

The number of risks that must be provided for and covered both through procedures and possible financing mechanisms is seemingly unlimited. Performing a vulnerability assessment and planning for the most likely scenarios to occur make selecting the best option more manageable.

Controls that a medical practice puts in place to reduce risk must be continually monitored to see if they are succeeding in reducing the risk. As new controls are implemented, the healthcare executive or risk manager needs to look at each risk and evaluate it. This is an ongoing process that will help determine if controls that are put into place are effective at reducing the risk. Audits are another way to determine if a risk control is effective. Audits are potent tools to use in areas such as staff training. An audit can be performed to see if the safety training for all required users of a piece of equipment has proven effective, for example.

Once a method of loss control is chosen, the tendency is to be so hopeful it works that signs of it not working are ignored. Regular monitoring and reevaluation of all loss control methods are therefore a crucial component of risk management. Standardized times should be scheduled for review of written policies and procedures, as well as actual processes performed in the organization. This ensures that the organization regularly updates all aspects of its risk management program.

1.2 Adverse Events

Medical errors fall into four categories, according to the Institute of Medicine: diagnostic, treatment, preventive, and other.[8]

Figure 5.1

Types of Errors

Diagnostic	Treatment
Error of delay in diagnosis Failure to employ indicated tests Use of outmoded tests or therapy Failure to act on results of monitoring or testing	Error in performance of an operation, procedure, or test Error in administering treatment Error in the dose or method of using a drug Avoidable delay in treatment or in responding to an abnormal test Inappropriate care
Preventive	**Other**
Failure to provide prophylactic treatment Inadequate monitoring or follow-up of treatment	Failure of communication Equipment failure Other system failure

Medical practices must have a plan in place to address any medical errors that may occur. All employees that play a part in patient care must be trained and know how to execute that plan when an error occurs. The plan should include these items, among others:

- How to identify medical errors
- How to report medical errors, including their documentation
- Who within the medical practice must be notified
- Steps for finding the cause of the error
- Steps for reviewing the error
- Steps for making changes, if needed, to prevent the error's recurrence
- Initiating risk-reduction strategies
- Ongoing training for all staff members

Safety is a broad term that encompasses many things. For medical practices, it can fall into two main categories: patient safety and employee safety. Both are important and must be considered.

A disaster is an event that makes normal functions impossible. Disasters can be natural or human-made. Examples of natural disasters include the destruction caused by Hurricane Katrina, the subsequent flooding of New Orleans in 2005, and the Arizona wildfires in the spring of 2006. Human-made disasters can be work stoppages, such as transit strikes in Philadelphia and New York, or the destruction caused by terrorist attacks on the World Trade Center in 2001.

Losses stemming from natural disasters provide examples of the variety needed in loss control methods.

Although there is much to be learned from the communication among various agencies, the military, and first responders, many aspects of an emergency plan may not go far enough to react adequately to different disasters.

In addition to natural and human-made disasters, increasing attention is being paid to the threat of an infectious disease pandemic. Medical practices should review disaster preparedness protocols and procedures in their organizations and communities to be current on the incorporation of pandemic preparedness into emergency management procedures, and what their own roles and responsibilities would be.

The COVID-19 pandemic of 2020 has made it clear how important it is for the medical community to be prepared for this type of emergency, both in protecting healthcare employees and preparing to treat large numbers of infected patients.

The Department of Health and Human Services and the Centers for Disease Control and Prevention (CDC) publish a number of resources specifically targeted to help medical offices and ambulatory clinics assess and improve their preparedness for responding to pandemics. Medical practices may find that they need to adapt the information and checklists to meet their unique needs.

According to the CDC, medical offices should develop a structure for planning and decision-making. The structure should include a planning committee with representation from both clinical staff (physicians, nurses, and ancillary personnel) and administrative staff, (healthcare executive and support staff), as well as the input of an environmental specialist, if possible. One person in the organization, such as the healthcare executive, should be assigned responsibility for coordinating preparedness planning for the practice. A point of contact (either someone in the clinic or an outside consultant) should be responsible for answering questions and/or providing consultation on infection control to prevent transmission of communicable diseases. The organizational structure should be described in a written plan.

The plan developed for the practice should be consistent with its existing emergency and disaster plans and with community response plans. No loss control mechanism should be selected without full consideration of the influence of local, cultural and environmental conditions on the potential for failure.

To protect the medical group's employees in times of emergency, it is important to create disaster plans. Most buildings have fire escape routes posted on the walls, lighted exit signs, and ceiling sprinkler systems. However, these precautions do not protect human life unless specific guidelines and drills are laid out, communicated to all employees, and practiced on a regular basis.

Policies should be in place directing supervisors and employees on how to handle emergency situations. Every employee should be notified about all emergency and disaster guidelines during orientation. Drills should be practiced at least once a year, and more frequently if possible. The policies should also direct employees on how to help patients and visitors reach safety.

Different geographic regions have different threats in terms of natural disasters. In California, for example, an earthquake emergency plan should be drafted to protect employees. Midwestern states should have tornado drills. Hurricane-prone areas should have evacuation plans in place for hurricanes and tropical storms. Every organization should promote "Be Prepared" for disaster programs so employees have emergency provisions and plans for their homes and families.

There are numerous websites, articles, and textbooks that document how to prepare a disaster recovery and business continuity plan. The best practices have been pulled together and refined to make them workable in a medical practice environment.

Here are four keys to disaster management:

1. Disaster preparedness: Are you ready for different scenarios that can affect the services you deliver? Have you performed a risk assessment, developed communication strategies, trained management and staff, and performed mock simulations?
2. Disaster response: Do you have a strategy for responding to the crisis, including communicating with patients and the community? This includes managing written, verbal, and social media communication.
3. Post-disaster recovery: Can you perform an impact assessment, including communicating with your key stakeholders, determining the effect of events on your community, and identifying strategies for repairing or restoring your reputation?
4. Debriefing: After the disaster, be certain to meet with your leadership team and board to discuss the disaster and how you handled each step of the process, and then fine-tune your plan for future unplanned events.

Taking the time to develop or refine your plans for responding to a crisis will save you and your organization time and money — and may save your reputation.

When performing a risk assessment, be sure to consider how the threat might affect the practice, as well as the likelihood of the threat.

Internal Control: Guidance for Directors on the Combined Code (also known as the Turnbull Report), published by the Internal Central Working Party of the Institute of Chartered Accountants in England and Wales, provides guidance on the implementation of internal controls, enabling companies to identify and respond to changing risks, both internal and external. The corporate governance codes recommended in this report published in 1999 are now being established worldwide.[9]

These codes help examine the financial, business, compliance, and operational areas of the business and rank the potential risks as high impact/high likelihood, high impact/low likelihood, low impact/high likelihood, and low impact/low likelihood. Ranking the perceived risks using this methodology prioritizes time and effort spent on projects, with potentially significant impacts for medical practices. It is also possible that the final plan may consist of a number of smaller plans, allowing several issues to be addressed once and inserted into various disaster recovery plan scenarios.

In addition to reviewing potential risks, it is also imperative to look at key performance indicators: the people, knowledge, and equipment that allow a practice to function each day. Without all three elements, the practice cannot function at its optimum level.

The most effective method of gathering critical information is usually with a survey, followed by a group meeting across all functions. This allows personnel to own a process, recognize the impact of a disaster on the individual department or function, and agree to the steps that need to be taken to get the functions back online.

During the discussions of impact analysis, the question of moving to an alternate site may arise. Disaster recovery plans refer to sites as hot, warm, and cold. A *hot site* is one that is a total standby environment. Unless the practice has an office in another location, on a different power grid and serviced by a different telephone provider, the expense of maintaining this type of site would be prohibitive. A *warm site* is a standby environment lacking only those requirements that can be provided quickly. For example, if there is a loss of power to one area of the building and a conference room is set up with additional phone and computer cabling powered by a generator, it could be used in this emergency situation. A *cold site* is a standby location without any hardware available. Without the luxury of having a backup office as a substitute, smaller practices would be forced to a cold site if access to the office is prohibited for any period of time.

Once the impact analysis is completed and there is a clearer understanding of the practice's critical processes, the strategy and contingency plan for getting these functions back online should be developed. The plan must clearly identify the tasks that need to be accomplished, along with the timeline for progress. It is also imperative that personnel responsible for these tasks be identified, as well as the location(s) to be used, that is, alternate office, home, cold site, and so forth.

This plan must be as detailed as possible if it is to be effective. Sit at a desk with only a computer and a phone and attempt to do a day's work. Within a short time, you recognize the little things that are used every day and taken for granted, such as printers, staplers, pens, pencils, sticky notes, and so on.

The methods and procedures for bringing back critical processes must be documented in the event the persons responsible have been adversely affected by the disaster and are unable to complete their tasks. The plan should cover the possibility that personnel may have other commitments if the disaster is wide ranging. They may have friends and family affected by the disaster or they may be responsible for the care of young children or elderly, sick relatives. If staff members have no access to money or transportation, they may be unable to get to work to assist with disaster recovery efforts.

After the plan has been developed, it is critical that it be tested. The testing is often the most difficult part of the planning process. Most experts in the field recommend testing parts of the plan, in short intervals, in case of plan failure. The only time a full-scale disaster drill should be called is when one is assured that all elements will function perfectly.

After reviewing the outline for developing a disaster recovery plan, look at critical processes that would be similar in almost all medical office practices, regardless of size or specialty. These processes include evacuation, communication, finances, insurance claims, human resources, clinical concerns, servers and information systems, telecommunications, and the physical plant.

If the building is unsafe due to fire, loss of electrical power, or any other reason, there should be a plan to safely evacuate staff, patients, and visitors. If the practice will not be able to access the premises for a period of time, all deposits and mail containing checks should be removed at the time of the evacuation, along with current encounters and chart notes.

If time allows, the servers should be powered down, and phones forwarded to a remote answering service. The person designated as the team leader for an evacuation should check the premises to ensure that all patients, visitors, and staff have departed. The staff should meet at a predetermined area to ensure that all employees have evacuated and can be accounted for.

Lines of communication must be set up with staff, patients, and vendors as soon as possible after a disaster. The healthcare executive or designee should have an employee contact list with home and cellular telephone numbers, as well as email addresses. If an employee is hurt during an evacuation, the practice will need emergency contact information readily available.

Cloud-based storage can be used to keep this information encrypted off-site for easy access after an emergency if the office computer is now unavailable.

Healthcare executives must have a process to contact patients. This includes a plan to have access to off-site backup data for patient names and phone numbers. An answering service acting as a backup call center can be a good solution if the office is inaccessible.

The practice must also contact vendors to let them know of the emergency and perhaps place orders for replacement equipment. Again, these numbers need to be stored off-site. In addition, account numbers, passwords, and other essential information must be available to the healthcare executive in case of an emergency.

Payroll must still be processed. Business interruption insurance is an excellent strategy to cover employment issues such as payroll and health insurance coverage. A prepared healthcare executive will make sure this insurance will cover the practice for an adequate time.

Vital practice information, such as managed care contracts, particularly those with carve-out reimbursements, must be accessible from an off-site facility. Contact information must be available so that payers can be alerted, which can help the practice avoid denials caused by late filing during this emergency period.

Information regarding the practice's insurance carriers must be available off-site. Commercial insurance covers buildings and contents, whereas business interruption insurance is meant to cover the incremental costs incurred during dislocation. Business interruption insurance does not cover the full cost of getting the practice back to normal working conditions. When formulating a disaster recovery plan, the healthcare executive should meet with the insurance carriers and discuss their requirements for damage documentation, their response times, and any policy limitations.

The needs of staff members must be reviewed and addressed as part of any successful disaster recovery plan. If the disaster has affected a wide area or a significant transportation route, employee issues will need to be resolved. Without alternate routes, employees may be unable to reach the worksite.

Most important for handling human resource issues during a time of disaster is to communicate, plan ahead, and involve the entire staff.

Information systems is the one area of disaster recovery that most practices have already addressed. Daily backups and redundant systems are standard procedure in today's practices. Employees working in remote locations should have the ability to access the practice network to allow certain employees, such as billers, to work from home for a period of time if the facility is not available.

Practices that use an application service provider (ASP) may have access to their data more quickly because the data and servers are off-site and possibly outside of the affected disaster area. However, it is important to investigate the ASP's disaster plans and ensure access to the medical practice data if they have a disruptive event at the vendor's site.

Consider the value of having the practice's answering service or call center located on a different power grid and telephone service area. The call center might still be functional and able to handle the practice's call volume. The call center must have its own disaster recovery plan, which should be reviewed by the practice.

If systems are up and running, but access to the site is being denied, the message system can be programmed remotely to alert patients of the office problem and options for follow-up.

When the practice can gain access to the physical plant, the first priority is to contain the damage. Save everything that can be salvaged, tested, or restored, and keep the damaged equipment for the adjustor to review. Maintain an up-to-date fixed inventory list and keep the list accessible remotely. The age and purchase price of the destroyed equipment will need to be documented. Copies of receipts and purchase records will speed the turnaround time on claims.

As part of the recovery plans, research vendors that can respond quickly to assess and contain fire and water damage. Keep the contact names and information for insurance claims. Although items may look unrecoverable, salvage must be started immediately to prevent rust, corrosion, and mold.

Keep a contact list of all vendors and make video or photo records of the damage incurred. Contact the practice insurance carrier immediately to perform a damage assessment. It may be quicker to replace equipment instead of restoring, but it's usually more expensive. Restoring avoids capital expenditure and improves cash flow.

After the critical processes for the practice have been established, the next step is to determine how quickly these need to be up and running. First, determine the:

- Maximum tolerable downtime, which is the maximum time an organization can tolerate being closed

- Recovery time objective, which is the time available to recover
- Recovery point objective (RPO), which is the extent of data lost
- Work recovery time (WRT), which is the time available to recover data

Critical process time frames are usually set at:

- Twenty-four hours
- Three to five days
- One to two weeks
- One to two months

Along with detailing the time frames to get processes up and running, it is critical that the healthcare executive determine when staff members should return to work. Time frames should be set for when the practice's billing, administrative, clinical, and ancillary staff should return.

1.3 Internal Controls and Audits

Internal controls and audits are not just recommended as part of a risk and compliance program, they are required. Any medical practice that treats patients using Medicare and Medicaid is required to maintain internal control measures and perform periodic audits to ensure patient safety and quality of care. Internal controls should include those for:

- Pharmaceutical compliance and tracking
- Temperature and autoclave logs
- Cleaning requirements and logging
- Prescription drug monitoring program

Laws and their interpretation are complex. It may be more common to be in violation of a legal nuance than to be certain that you comply. Furthermore, the rapid proliferation of legislation at all levels of government, coupled with a focus on patient safety and patient rights, means it is possible for statutes in the same jurisdiction to conflict. Even within state laws, conflict can exist, or be perceived to exist, when interpreted by different legal entities.

It is essential for the healthcare executive with risk management responsibility to have a relationship with a respected, ethical, and efficient law firm. The medical group needs an attorney familiar with general legal principles and general business issues. This may be an attorney who serves as the central point for ensuring there are no conflicts among the specialists.

This attorney may also be the one who watches out for the best interests of the organization in a general way, keeping an eye on the changes in local, state, or federal law that may be of interest to the organization.

In addition, the medical practice should engage attorneys specifically trained in healthcare and environmental issues, medical malpractice, compliance, employment, real estate, human resource, and contract law. (Some attorneys may specialize in more than one of these areas.) The healthcare executive should work with each of these specialists and have them coordinate with one another to ensure that conflicting perspectives will not create additional risk exposure for the practice.

1.4 Media Relations

Most experts agree that the most effective way to maintain a positive public image is to be transparent in all things, including communication. When it comes to risk and compliance, the compliance plan should include a plan for how to communicate in the event of a medical error or adverse event, and who will be doing the communicating.

The adverse event, disaster communication, or crisis communication plan can help your hospital or medical practice be prepared for the emergency and potential negative press.

Keep the following communication tips in mind:

Don't panic: Unfortunately, when faced with a crisis, the first instinct of many healthcare executives and other medical leadership is to hide and hope it goes away. Others get defensive. Obviously, none of these responses is very smart. Instead, you can plan ahead. A good crisis communications plan anticipates potential problems and develops a response for each scenario. It designates roles and responsibilities for each member of the crisis team, identifies a primary spokesperson, and establishes a command center where accurate information can be managed and delivered at specified times through specific channels, such as your website, social media, or a media briefing.

Follow the CAP formula: CAP stands for compassion, action, and perspective. Keeping those principles at the forefront during a crisis can help prevent more problems:

Compassion: The most important part of your response is to show compassion to the public. For example, "Our top priority is the safety of our patients and staff. We've established a 24-hour hotline where patients and family members can get information and we've arranged counseling for our employees." Provide accurate, honest information as quickly as possible. Explain what you know so far by sticking to the facts. Never speculate, and make sure to focus on public benefits instead of the practice's problems. Speak with one consistent voice.

Action: Explain what you are doing to fix the problem and make sure that it does not happen again. For example, "We are reviewing all our safety and hiring procedures to make sure that our security and screening processes are the best they can be."

Perspective: Use your history to your advantage, for example, "We've been a part of this community for 50 years. Nothing like this has ever happened, and we are doing everything we can to make sure this is an isolated incident and that it never happens again."

It's vital to establish and maintain good relationships with local media and your patients. It can help you mitigate the potential damage by making it more likely that the reporter and the public will give you the benefit of the doubt. Once you get that opportunity, don't waste it. Make sure you adhere to the following guidelines:

- Communicate openly, honestly, factually, and compassionately.
- Keep your cool. Don't get baited into a confrontation.
- Ask the reporter for an opportunity to convey your point of view. When needed, ask for a meeting to tell your side of the story.
- Avoid saying "no comment." It sounds like you have something to hide. If you don't know the answer, tell reporters you will find out and get back to them. If your lawyer recommends not answering, find a way to respond without giving your lawyer a heart attack.
- Stay on message. Create three key messages and stick to them as much as possible. "We are devastated that this happened." "We are doing everything we can to fix the problem." "This is an isolated incident, and we are doing everything in our power to make sure it will never happen again." Express your key points and repeat them as often as you can without sounding like a robot.

SAMPLE QUESTIONS

1. What is loss control?

A. Using selected techniques, including financing, for failed control of losses

B. The identification and analysis of exposures

C. The continuous observation of selected methods for controlling losses for potential improvement

D. A risk management technique that seeks to reduce the possibility that a loss will occur and reduce the severity of those that do occur

2. Which sentence about natural disasters is true?

A. Different geographic regions have different threats in terms of natural disasters

B. There is an equal chance that all natural disasters will occur

C. Organizations should have a plan in place for all natural disasters

D. Organizations should only have a plan in place for natural disasters

Answers: 1-D, 2-A

TASK 2: COMPLIANCE WITH APPLICABLE LAWS AND REGULATIONS

When most practices think of compliance, laws and regulations are at the forefront of their minds, and with good reason. The healthcare industry is heavily regulated to ensure the safety of patient care. In addition to these laws and regulations, practices have special concerns when it comes to employee safety. Practices often must deal with hazardous waste of all kinds, as well as safe handling of sharps and pharmaceuticals. However, compliance with all federal, state, and local laws and regulations must be an integral part of a medical practice's compliance plan.

KEY TERMS

OIG: U.S. Department of Health, Office of Inspector General.

PHI: Protected health information.

The OIG developed separate compliance guidelines for individual and small group physician practices, and offers these seven components for the development of a sound compliance program:[10]

- Conduct internal monitoring and audits
- Implement compliance and practice standards
- Have a designated compliance officer or person
- Provide appropriate training and education
- Respond appropriately to any offenses that are detected, and take steps to correct them
- Develop and maintain open lines of communication
- Develop practice compliance guidelines and enforce them

2.1 Federal and State Requirements and Reporting

Many federal, state, and local laws and regulations affect healthcare organizations.

The Health Insurance Portability and Accountability Act of 1996 (HIPAA) is a law enacted to protect the health information of patients, combat waste, fraud, and abuse in health insurance and delivery, and simplify the administration of health insurance. HIPPA covers both individuals and organizations. Those who must comply with HIPAA are often called HIPAA-covered entities. The Department of Health and Human Services (HSS) is the government agency that administers HIPAA. HHS recognized that electronic health records might pose risks to privacy of patients, so HIPAA was updated in 2000 and again in 2002 to include a privacy rule update. In 2003, a security rule was also added to HIPAA.

Medical practices must comply with HIPAA when gathering, storing, and communicating patients' personal information, as well as individually identifiable health information. HIPAA ensures that all U.S. citizens have the civil right to access their health information and that their health information is protected from others gaining access. The primary sections of HIPAA that practices should know and understand are:

- Privacy
- Security
- Administrative Simplification
- Compliance and Enforcement
- Patient Safety

Privacy Rule standards specify how covered health information (protected health information, or PHI) can be used for treatment and billing of patients, as well as how it should be protected. HIPAA's goal is to protect health information while also ensuring that information necessary for treating patients flows efficiently among providers and insurers.

The Security Rule established a set of standards intended to protect health information when it is being kept or communicated in electronic form. All of the standards in the Privacy Rule apply. The Security Rule focuses its standards on the storage and communication of electronic patient records and information. Just as it did with the Privacy Rule, the Office of Civil Rights (OCR) is responsible for enforcing the Security Rule and imposing penalties on any practice that violates it.

One of the Security Rule's primary objectives is to protect patients' health information while at the same time allowing practices to adopt new technologies that can improve patient care quality and efficiency.

All medical practices that transmit health information or conduct healthcare transactions in electronic form are subject to the Security Rule. The Security Rule also applies to a medical practice's business associates, as defined by the Privacy Rule.

The Security Rule focuses on and protects a specific subset of information covered by the Privacy Rule, which is all individually identifiable health information a practice creates, receives, maintains, or transmits in electronic form. This is called electronic protected health information under the Security Rule, or e-PHI. The Security Rule does not apply to PHI transmitted orally or in writing.

The Security Rule states that practices must:

- Ensure that all patient e-PHI created, received, stored, or communicated by the practice is kept confidential, its integrity remains intact, and it is available when requested or needed
- Ensure that the practice takes the steps necessary to identify and protect e-PHI from security threats or corruption of the information
- Ensure the practice protects e-PHI from reasonably anticipated disclosures of information that violate HIPAA regulation
- Ensure the practice gains workforce compliance with the Security Rule (i.e., all employees are aware of regulations and practice policies and procedures to ensure compliance)

The Center for Medicaid/Medicare Services (CMS) is a division of the U.S. Department Health and Human Services. Among other things, CMS provides oversight, guidance, and enforcement of Medicaid and Medicare programs and efforts to prevent fraud, waste, and abuse in these programs, primarily through the Centers for Program Integrity (CPI). CMS provides resources for providers and states. In its compliance program your practice should include the fraud, waste, and abuse regulations and ensure employees know them.

The Occupational Safety and Health Administration (OSHA), a division of the U.S. Department of Labor, is responsible for ensuring safe working conditions for the nation's employees. It does this by publishing and enforcing standards and guidelines. The nature of medical practices means employees can be exposed to additional health and safety risks, so it is especially important that practices are aware of and follow all OSHA standards. Whether your medical practice has two or 200 employees, it must follow most OSHA standards. Failing to comply with OSHA standards could cost your practice money in fines, as well as adversely affect employee health and safety.

Primary OSHA standards and regulations your practice must comply with include those concerning:

- Bloodborne pathogens
- Hazard communication
- Ionizing radiation
- Exit routes
- Emergency action plans
- Electrical standards
- OSHA poster display
- Reporting violations

OSHA requires that every employer covered by the law provide employees with a place of employment that is free from recognized hazards to life or health. The act further provides that employees comply with all standards, rules, regulations, and orders issued by the employers to comply with the law.

Most small medical groups choose to select an individual to be responsible for safety in the workplace. Larger medical practices may appoint a safety officer for this role. Regardless of the organization's size, management should develop a comprehensive safety program suited to the group's particular needs and enforced by the compliance or safety officer.

Much of safety and health compliance relies on providing educational safety and health training programs. Training programs must be in place and mandatory for all employees. A safety committee responsible for all safety and health programs and safety incentive programs are other ways to ensure compliance with regulations. Employees who do not follow the safety policies should be properly disciplined to ensure that safety regulations are followed.

Other areas to consider in the safety policy are:

- On-the-job injuries
- Accident and injury reports
- Medical emergencies
- Posting of emergency information
- Evacuation plan
- First aid equipment
- Weather-related alerts
- Care and use of equipment
- Violence and terrorism threats
- Bomb threats
- Protective clothing
- Safety inspections
- Reporting of unsafe conditions
- Firearms
- Safety designated areas
- Safety suggestions
- Incentive award programs

These 10 tips will help enforce OSHA standards in a group practice. These tips are directed to the OSHA safety manager at the practice:

1. Add OSHA managerial duties to the OSHA safety manager's job description. The practice's OSHA safety officer needs time to accomplish those duties, so it's important that the job description includes OSHA responsibilities.
2. Make sure everyone understands who wears the OSHA hat. Encourage staff to bring safety concerns to that person's attention and encourage that person to be the go-to person for safety advice and leadership.
3. Take all complaints seriously, with an open door and open mind to all safety concerns. Employees often call OSHA when they believe management isn't listening. Minor issues need to be handled before they escalate into major problems.
4. Document everything. At inspection or incident investigation time, if it wasn't written down, it didn't happen.
5. Consider safety a value rather than a priority. Business priorities change over time, but values endure. Since the needs of the moment determine business priorities, safety might not always hold a place at the top of the list.
6. Make safety compliance a requirement in each employee's job description. Discipline employees who purposely don't comply. First, document

the problem. Then speak with the employee. If the problem persists, document the incident and inform the supervisor. For serious cases, approach senior management and consider termination.

7. Manage by walking around. This well-known approach lets the safety officer learn if employees merely give lip service to OSHA regulations.
8. Make annual OSHA training applicable to your practice. Preview videos and identify areas where you can use examples from your practice to reinforce the education. Keep employees involved; have them voice opinions or demonstrate techniques.
9. Keep your cool. Manage OSHA tasks using monthly and annual checklists to organize the safety officer's duties. Listen to employee concerns, but don't take safety-related criticisms personally.
10. Remind organizational leaders of the benefits of OSHA compliance. Part of managing your practice's OSHA safety program is quantifying its contributions, which are fewer injuries, less downtime, reduced worker compensation claims, and improved employee morale.

Information and training are the core elements of a hazard communication program, which is intended to prevent illness or injury from chemical exposure. Training should include education about the HCS, hazardous properties of all chemicals in the workplace, and methods of protection to ensure a safe work environment. Each employee should comprehend and understand the risks associated with any potential exposure. The hazard communication program is a written plan that describes how an employer will implement and comply with the HCS. This plan will be the initial focus of an investigation if an OSHA compliance officer conducts an inspection. It should include a complete list of all potentially hazardous chemicals in the workplace, corresponding SDSs, how the SDSs will be maintained and accessed, and documentation of training and education on labeling use and SDSs.

Each employer must have a designated OSHA compliance officer who is responsible for maintaining an up-to-date list of all hazardous chemicals in the workplace and current SDSs on each of the chemicals in the office. The compliance officer should also determine if the chemical containers are properly labeled and updated.

Employees should know where to access safety data sheets (SDSs) in the workplace. Detailed procedures for purchasing, receiving, storing, and handling chemicals should be readily available. When a new chemical is introduced in the workplace, employees should be educated about the chemical before it is used.

EXHIBIT 5.1

Hazard Communication Standard Compliance Checklist[11]

- ☐ Obtain a copy of the rule
- ☐ Read and understand the requirements
- ☐ Assign responsibility for tasks
- ☐ Prepare an inventory of chemicals
- ☐ Ensure that containers are labeled
- ☐ Obtain a safety data sheet for each chemical
- ☐ Prepare a written program
- ☐ Make safety data sheets available to employees
- ☐ Conduct employee training
- ☐ Establish procedures to maintain the current program
- ☐ Establish procedures to evaluate effectiveness of the program

Employee training is imperative. Training should create knowledge of materials and equipment, the known and potential hazards that may exist in the workplace, and how to control or minimize those hazards. No employee should undertake a job until they have been properly trained to perform the duties of the job, nor undertake a job that appears unsafe or in which potential hazards have not been minimized.

All new employees should receive training on the general standards of the facility (e.g., fire and evacuation procedures) and job-specific hazards as a part of their orientation. Staff should have additional training when changes in the work environment alter potential or actual safety hazards. Annual training should be provided on all aspects of the safety compliance program. Documentation of this training should include a list with signatures of the employees present, the date, the type of training, the subjects covered in the training, the person performing the training, and the trainer's credentials.

CMS oversees and enforces laws and regulations intended to prevent fraud, waste, and abuse (FWA).

Fraud is defined as executing a scheme (directly or indirectly) or intentionally submitting false information to gain money or property from any healthcare benefit program.

Waste is defined as practices that result in unnecessary costs to the Medicare program. These practices could include overusing services or misusing resources. Waste is not considered a criminal practice.

Abuse occurs when the service provider (directly or indirectly) receives payments for services or items when it is not entitled to them.

The primary difference between abuse and fraud is that there is no intentionality with abuse — the service provider has not intentionally submitted false information.

The False Claims Act (FCA) was enacted during the Civil War when Congress feared that suppliers of goods to the Union Army were defrauding the government. The FCA has been updated and amended several times. Currently, the law states that any individual or entity who knowingly submits false claims to the government is liable to pay three times the government's cost (damages) plus a penalty. False claims can include those submitted to obtain property or payments or those made to avoid having to pay the government. To fall under this law, false claims are submitted knowingly.

The Health Care Fraud Statute also makes it illegal to make false claims against the government's healthcare benefit programs. Under this statute, any person or entity who knowingly or willingly tries to defraud a health benefit program is subject to pay a fine and/or serve up to 10 years in prison.

Criminal Health Care Fraud penalties can also be sought, especially when the false claims or violations result in death. In criminal fraud cases the penalty paid can be as much as $250,000 and result in imprisonment for up to 20 years.

The Anti-Kickback Statute is part of the Social Security Act. This statute makes it illegal to ask for, receive, or pay a kickback, bribe, or rebate for referring a patient or practice for services that are covered or reimbursed by a government health benefit program, including Medicare.

Similarly, the Stark Law regulations (I and II) prohibit referral by a provider to any entity in which the provider has a financial relationship. Known as the Ethics in Patient Referrals Act of 1989, Stark Law I was promulgated in an effort to deter referrals to substandard providers.

In addition to healthcare laws and regulations, medical practices also must comply with federal and state laws concerning labor and human resources. These laws include:

- The Fair Labor Standards Act
- Employee Retirement Income Security Act of 1974 (ERISA)
- Family Medical Leave Act of 1993 (FMLA)
- United Services Employment and Reemployment Act
- Federal Civil Rights Act
- Americans with Disabilities Act (ADA)
- ADA Amendments Act of 2008 (ADAA)
- Age Discrimination Employment Act
- Occupational Health and Safety Act (1970)
- Equal Pay Act
- National Labor Relations Act
- Pregnancy Discrimination Act

CMS, as part of its efforts to prevent fraud, waste, and abuse, requires all practices to report any overpayments they receive from the Medicare or

Medicaid system within 60 days of their occurrence. They are also required to return that overpayment. Practices are also required to look at all payments they have received as far back as the past six years to ensure no overpayments have been made.[12]

The Office for Civil Rights (OCR) is responsible for enforcing the HIPAA Privacy and Security Rules. OCR accomplishes this by investigating complaints it receives.

OCR can only act on complaints that meet the following criteria:

- The alleged incident took place when the rules were in effect
- The complaint is filed against an organization that is mandated to comply with the rules
- The complaint must describe an incident that is in violation of the rules
- The complaint must be filed within 180 days of the person finding out about the incident

In cases that OCR investigates, it reviews all the information and then determines whether the organization did violate a privacy or security rule. If the evidence does indicate that the organization acted in violation of the rules, it will attempt to resolve the issue with the organization by doing one of the following:

- Asking for voluntary compliance
- Taking corrective action
- Creating a resolution agreement

If an organization named in a complaint does not act to resolve the matter in a way the OCR finds acceptable, the OCR may then decide to fine the organization, imposing what are called civil monetary penalties (CMPs). In the event that CMPs are charged, the organization is given the opportunity to request a hearing headed by an HHS administrative law judge.

Additionally, certain types of violations may be subject to criminal prosecution. The HHS describes three levels of criminal prosecution HHS may pursue for certain types of violations:

1. Misusing a unique health identifier may lead to a $25,000 fine and one year in prison
2. Obtaining information under a false pretense could lead to a $100,000 fine and five years in prison
3. If the intent of the organization named in the complaint was to sell or use PHI for personal gain or malicious harm, the fine could rise to $250,000 with a possible jail term of 10 years

In addition to third-party complaints, if an organization discovers a security breach in which health information was exposed, the organization must notify the Secretary of Health and Human Services. All notifications must be submitted to the Secretary using the web portal on the HHS website.

There are several types of breaches that can occur at any organization, but some of the more common ones are:

- Hacking/IT incident
- Improper disposal of paper records
- Loss of paper or e-PHI
- Theft of mobile devices and/or paper records

Practices should keep in mind that breaches can occur anywhere and at any time, including:

- Desktop, laptop and tablet computers
- Email that is unencrypted
- Electronic Medical Record (EMR)
- Network servers
- Smart phone
- Paper files

Two agencies are primarily responsible for regulating the protection of employees and patients from communicable diseases: OSHA and the CDC. OSHA focuses on protecting healthcare employees from contracting a communicable disease, and CDC focuses on preventing the spread of these diseases through actions such as quarantines and vaccinations.

OSHA regulations that medical practices should be sure to know and comply with include:

- Bloodborne Pathogen Standard
- Personal Protective Equipment Standard
- Respiratory Protection Standard
- TB Compliance Directive

CDC regulations or guidelines for medical practices include:

- Hand Hygiene in Healthcare Settings
- Guide to Infection Prevention for Outpatient Settings: Minimum Expectations for Safe Care
- Guideline for Disinfection and Sterilization in Healthcare Facilities, 2008

State guidelines may vary when it comes to communicable or infectious disease prevention. The COVID-19 pandemic created the need for additional precautions specific to this highly contagious disease. Medical practices should monitor CDC and OSHA standards daily during pandemic situations.

According to the OIG, the most important government acts, regulations and standards that must be part of a medical practice compliance program are:

- The Emergency Medical Treatment and Labor Act (EMTALA): This requires medical centers that provide emergency medical treatments to provide treatment to patients regardless of their ability to pay

- Clinical Laboratory Improvement Amendments (CLIA): The CLIA regulates all laboratory testing (except research) performed on humans in the United States
- Anti-kickback laws
- Research laws
- Stark Law

The Red Flags Rule is a regulatory code from the Federal Trade Commission (FTC). These are guidelines for helping all businesses, including medical practices, recognize when attempts at identity theft are occurring. It is part of the Fair Reporting Credit Act: Identity Theft Rules. Red flags are signs that identify theft is being attempted. The rules give businesses who provide credit for billing, as some practices do, these signs to watch for. Examples include:

- Personal identifying information is inconsistent with information from external sources
- The address does not match any address in the person's consumer report
- The social security number is shown as not issued yet or is on a list of numbers associated with people who have died
- The address given is fictitious, a mail drop, or prison

Because of vandalism, thefts, bomb scares, terrorism, and major incidences of workplace violence, securing your facility is important. For example, the theft of business equipment, especially small items, has greatly increased in recent years and is very costly to employers. The threat of computer hacking and viruses requires technological security precautions and thorough employee education.

Security programs involve taking precautionary measures to ensure adequate protection of the group practice's property and assets, as well as that of its employees and patients. A group practice's security needs vary depending on its location, the nature of its operations, and number of employees. Some large groups hire security consultants to develop, administer, and audit their security programs, but even the smallest practice needs to create, implement, and enforce written security policies.

Each medical practice has its own unique needs. A practice with a great deal of computer equipment might want or need a specific rider to cover that equipment. A practice that has a swimming pool to provide physical therapy needs specific coverage for that. In general, the following types of insurance account for the most common kinds of insurance coverage for a group medical practice:

- Professional liability (medical malpractice)
- General liability
- Property and casualty
- Cybersecurity insurance (either a specific rider on the general liability or through the malpractice carrier)
- Directors' and officers' liability for errors and omissions

- Workers' compensation (which is not an employee benefit, but a risk control coverage)
- Key person (in small practices)
- Employment liability
- Environmental
- Vehicle
- Helipad (if the organization has one)
- Business interruption

A skilled broker can also advise the client if self-insurance is in the client's best interest. Working with the broker and an actuary, the organization can conduct a feasibility study. Sometimes the practice will be approaching readiness for self-insurance but is not yet ready to "take the leap." A broker can design an interim short-term insurance program or stop-loss policy that will allow the practice to assume part of the risk before taking the plunge into full self-insurance.

Regardless of the type of vehicle selected to finance risk, the organization benefits from tight loss control processes. The temptation to diminish loss control when there is commercial insurance must be avoided. When the insurance market is tight and there is little competition for customers, those practices with the best loss records and the tightest loss control methods will be the ones with choices regarding an insurer.

Reduction of loss exposure is not just the job of the person with risk management responsibility. It requires commitment on the part of the board and administration to provide the necessary resources for loss control. It further requires that physicians understand the benefit of loss control methods to their practice and that time spent participating in risk management activities may mean less time spent defending their practice in lawsuits. Finally, all personnel must realize that risk management is the job of each person in the organization.

Although attributed to insurance, true risk management is about people, patients, and staff, as well as maintaining a fiscally viable organization so that the people who work there will continue to have a place to work and to serve others.

The primary goal of the ADA, as it applies to facilities, is to ensure that individuals with disabilities have safe and easy access, and can maneuver within a place of public accommodation. To comply with the ADA, a practice must address a host of physical design features. These include ensuring that doors are wide enough to allow for the passage of a wheelchair, providing restroom facilities that can be easily used by people with disabilities, and providing adequate designated handicapped parking.

The designated safety person in your practice should be familiar with Life Safety Codes. These codes were developed by the National Fire Prevention Association (NFPA) and were designed to minimize the possibility of fires, as well as their effects. The practice should plan to meet all applicable Life Safety Codes for their facilities and all employees should be trained on them. Life Safety Codes also address crowd safety and non-fire emergencies.

Private inurement refers to the practice of a person or people at a nonprofit organization using charitable funds for private gain. Examples include executives of nonprofit organizations using funds for personal travel, home remodeling, and car leases. Many organizations in the healthcare industry are nonprofit. It is important that all employees of these organizations recognize that private inurement is illegal and watch for signs that this may be happening. All nonprofit organizations should have safeguards in their accounting departments, as well as policies and procedures to ensure that funds cannot be used for personal purchases.

Healthcare organizations should also ensure that they comply with all federal, state, and local tax regulations. The best way to do this is to hire a tax specialist, either an in-house person or staff to handle the organization's tax requirements, or an outside tax service agency to handle them.

Some healthcare organizations and practices have a misconception that efforts to collect on past due accounts do not have to follow the same rules as any other debt collection efforts. This is certainly not the case. Any debt that is incurred by a person for personal reasons, and healthcare falls into this category, must meet consumer debt collection laws and regulations.

The Fair Debt Collection Practices Act applies to healthcare debt collection and addresses, among other issues:

- How collectors may find the location of the debtor
- Communication
- Harassment or abuse
- False or misleading representations
- Legal actions by debt collectors

2.2 Compliance Plans

Corporate compliance is an area that has confused many people because of the number and types of laws that are included in this diverse area. In its simplest terms, corporate compliance is the organization's program to ensure that it meets all relevant federal and state laws as well as the program requirements of federal, state, and private health plans. In actuality, a compliance program also includes the formula for executing and running a compliance program as defined by the U.S. Department of Health and Human Services, Office of Inspector General (OIG), and the requirements of agencies that monitor compliance in healthcare.

The OIG-recommended compliance program elements are based on the Federal Sentencing Guidelines.[13] The OIG believes that every hospital and integrated healthcare delivery system, regardless of size, location, or corporate structure, should apply all of the following elements, modified to fit its unique situation:

- Develop written standards of conduct (often referred to as a code of conduct)
- Provide continuing education to all staff members on these standards of conduct

Develop written policies and procedures to promote the organization's commitment to compliance (e.g., medical and business record policies, evaluation of managers on adherence to policies, and monitoring of necessity of care) and to address specific areas of potential fraud, including but not limited to:

- Incorrect reimbursement
- Record falsification
- Fraudulent billing and documentation practices
- Billing errors
- Inadequate documentation of care
- Continuation of unneeded or unauthorized care
- Inadequate patient information
- Client abuse
- Patient discrimination
- Inadequate safety plan for patients and staff
- Inappropriate acceptance of gifts

Different regulations and statutes apply to the retention of patient medical records and employee health or OSHA records. Patient medical records are generally retained in accordance with the statute of limitations for bringing malpractice action, as defined by the individual state. Employee records must be retained in accordance with the type of employee health services provided on-site. For both types of records, the medical practice should confer with counsel familiar with the applicable statutes.

The primary responsibility for ensuring proper storage and retention should include a designated backup should the process owner (e.g., the healthcare executive) be unavailable. The plan should also include a loss control process for electronic backup of important documents.

Record retention is a critical issue in group practices. There are several medical practice concerns as well as legal issues to consider when retaining records. Laws regarding recordkeeping vary from state to state. Policies need to be developed to clearly indicate:

- Type of record, such as financial, employee, property, tax returns, medical record, or other
- Whether the record is electronic or paper
- Location of the record
- How long it should be retained
- Who is authorized to order record destruction
- Who should have access to records

Despite being modern tools, electronic records are not indestructible. In addition to the safeguards of physical separation and redundancy of files, a variety of individuals should have access to the files. It is often advisable to keep the source documents (such as paper forms) for a period of time commensurate with state regulation. Transcription errors, disputes about the validity of the documentation, and allegations of misrepresentation are likely to arise early in the life of a document. Historical documents provide a framework for decisions but may be called on more rarely in litigation.

Compliance audits of all applicable departments and areas should be done at least annually, or more frequently, when appropriate. Quarterly or randomized audits may be necessary if prior audits have detected systemic errors requiring more frequent monitoring.

When deficiencies or errors are detected in internal or external audits, document the action plan with appropriate follow-up actions, including the project review and end date. A log with compliance issues should be maintained and the healthcare executive should work closely with appropriate departments to investigate any issues.

The investigation needs to be comprehensive, and each group should document the steps performed and support, defend, or remedy the actions associated with the claim. The compliance log helps ensure a level of consistency in handling situations and identifying trends. Any deficiency should be addressed with additional education and communication about the importance of compliance. The leadership team should share topics of concern, not specific cases, to illustrate to staff the organizational policies and procedures to avoid recurrence of violations resulting from misunderstanding or ignorance of the rules and standards.

The compliance plan or practice procedures and policies should indicate when employee retraining or disciplinary action is warranted, up to and including termination. A review may determine that the practice should report a single violation or a pattern of behavior to the applicable agency or authority. As an example, some medical practices have zero-tolerance policies when there is inappropriate access to patient medical records. Any access not related to a business purpose results in termination. In these practices, strong compliance commitments are explained during employee orientation and onboarding and reinforced with regular communication, training, and education.

The committee should continuously develop an education program that drills down to the physician and employee levels. The program should include information and training on job performance in compliance with practice standards, applicable regulations, and commitment to an effective compliance program. The OIG has created educational materials to explain federal laws on fraud, waste, and abuse, including a physician self-study booklet titled *A Roadmap for New Physicians*, with a companion Microsoft® PowerPoint presentation and speaker notes.[14] This presentation can be supplemented with customized training on compliance roles for physicians and staff.

Compliance with federal and state laws and regulations is everyone's responsibility. Whether it is the fiduciary responsibility for the board members or accuracy of claims by the billing staff, the commitment to compliance is organizational as well as individual. The compliance process is also dynamic and requires engagement to ensure that groups fulfill all the elements of an effective compliance program. By considering these suggestions, healthcare professionals demonstrate their commitment to corporate compliance.

SAMPLE QUESTIONS

1. **Which medical practice employee should be responsible for OSHA administration tasks?**

   A. Office manager

   B. Safety manager

   C. Lead physician

   D. All employees are responsible

2. **What are red flags?**

   A. Signs that OSHA standards have been violated

   B. Signs that OCR needs to be contacted

   C. Signs that identity theft is being attempted

   D. Signs that HIPAA violations have occurred

Answers: 1-B, 2-C

TASK 3: ACCREDITATION, CREDENTIALING, AND LICENSING (INDIVIDUALS AND ORGANIZATIONS)

Prior to officially joining any practice — and in many cases, prior to the interview — physicians will need to complete several credentialing processes. These steps are critical for many legal reasons.[15]

Laws in every state and the District of Columbia establish provider licensure requirements for persons practicing medicine. Some jurisdictions prohibit, either through explicit statements in their medical practice acts or through case law, the corporate practice of medicine. This doctrine generally forbids physicians from practicing medicine on behalf of, or in concert with, any organization other than a professional services corporation (or similar corporate entity) for the practice of medicine. In some states, similar limitations are also imposed, to a greater or lesser degree, on other licensed healthcare professionals (e.g., psychologists) delivering services in a corporate setting.

Many states have eased up on this strict prohibition to allow nonprofit hospital service corporations, health maintenance organizations, and certain other enterprises to employ physicians.

To meet these legal requirements, providers and their healthcare executives must take many credentialing steps, some of which are required before physicians can legally practice medicine. These requirements include obtaining the following:

- Employer identification number
- State tax identification number
- Medical license for every state in which the provider plans to practice
- Drug Enforcement Administration (DEA) permit
- Hospital privileges
- Payer credentialing after receiving state license and DEA clearance
- Medicare and/or Medicaid credentialing

Credentialing may take many months, and some employers will not allow a new provider to begin employment until the provider has received a certificate of completion from residency and all credentialing is complete.

Every physician must have a state license and a DEA permit to practice medicine. Also, most practices will not allow a new physician to begin work until the insurance carriers, including Medicare and Medicaid, have credentialed the physician. After the physician has been credentialed, they can bill for and receive reimbursement for services rendered.

A physician's training license is not a state license. Physicians must apply for licensure in every state in which they wish to practice. If your group practice has a satellite office in a neighboring state, confirm that the state will allow doctors to practice if they're licensed in a neighboring state and working for an organization with sites in both states.

Insurance carriers also have a separate process for providers to be credentialed in their system. This credentialing is necessary in order for the practice to be reimbursed by the insurance company and is separate from credentialing for practice privileges. Each insurance company contracts with a provider and has its own application process. This can take three to six months. Thus, each new provider can face a six- to nine-month process to acquire necessary credentials.

For organizations and facilities, the primary accrediting bodies are the Joint Commission on Accreditation of Healthcare Organizations and the Accreditation Association for Ambulatory Health Care. When pursuing accreditation, a practice or healthcare facility should undergo a rigorous multi-day evaluation that addresses all aspects of the operation of the organization and the medical treatment that is being provided. Within this accreditation process, an organization can expect that evaluations of the following areas will take place:

- Governing bylaws
- Safety and health procedures
- Facility design and safety
- Chart documentation
- Human resources
- Quality assurance reviews
- Physician and staff credentialing

The development, implementation, and adherence to documented policies and procedures that delineate and govern the day-to-day operations of the practice are critical to the successful completion of the accreditation process. This in-depth evaluation is repeated, normally on a three-year cycle, to ensure that the findings of both the initial and subsequent evaluations are still within the expected values that earned the organization its original accreditation.

In addition to the professional credentialing organizations previously discussed, physicians are also credentialed by licensed healthcare facilities (e.g., hospitals and nursing homes) and by commercial and noncommercial insurance carriers. Each organization has its own policies and procedures for credentialing providers and confirming and updating those credentials. Each accredited entity has its own regulations that must be followed by the provider, such as proof of advanced life support training or tuberculosis screening.

To properly and effectively manage the myriad regulations, licenses, and credentialing requirements of its healthcare providers, it is advantageous for the practice to develop a database that reflects and summarizes all of the requirements so the practice's leadership can easily identify areas of conflict or areas where information requires updating.

There are different types of medical malpractice insurance. Here are the most common types along with what they entail:[16]

1. Claims-based: A claims-based or claims-made policy will only provide coverage if the policy was in effect when the incident took place and the lawsuit was filed. This means a long-term policy.

2. Occurrence-based: An occurrence-based policy provides coverage if the policy was in effect when the incident took place, even if it is no longer in effect. This is usually a more expensive policy.
3. Malpractice tail insurance: Tail insurance is usually purchased by physicians when a claims-based policy has lapsed, and a new policy will not cover incidents that took place during the previous time period.[17]

In general, medical malpractice insurance is a must-have for any physician, but as many healthcare executives know, higher coverage limits aren't necessarily a good thing. Experts say that high limits can lead to plaintiffs seeking higher judgments. Because tort reform caps on the amount plaintiffs can be awarded vary from state to state, bigger limits aren't always better.

Eight considerations when choosing the level of medical malpractice insurance are:

1. Understand hospital credentialing and managed care plan requirements
2. Know your specialty requirements; certain specialties might need to carry higher insurance limits than others
3. Consider what might happen if a judgment in excess of coverage limits is granted
4. Find an insurance broker who's familiar with malpractice insurance in your state
5. Organizational structure can also offer you some protection; limited liability companies (LLCs) and limited liability partnerships, for example, might give your organization an advantage when it comes to malpractice suits
6. Be very familiar with the providers in the practice before purchasing insurance
7. Use networking to reach out to other executives or managers in your region to determine their experience with specific insurance companies
8. Healthcare executives should also familiarize themselves with different types of malpractice coverage, such as tail coverage, claims-made versus occurrence-made malpractice insurance, and more

Ongoing compliance must be a part of the day-to-day operation of the practice. Committee meetings, code blue and disaster drills, ongoing staff training, organization of human resource and administrative documents, quality control studies, and ongoing review are all items that become part of the daily, weekly, and monthly routine. Every aspect of the practice is reviewed during the accreditation process. Accreditation offers the opportunity for in-depth analysis of operations. A key individual on staff who is familiar with all departments, skilled at organization, capable with computer documentation, and endlessly patient is vital to successful compliance.

SAMPLE QUESTIONS

1. **What two types of licensure must a physician have before they may practice medicine?**

   A. State license and malpractice insurance

   B. Malpractice insurance and a driver's license

   C. State license and a driver's license

   D. State license and a DEA permit to practice medicine

2. **Which type of malpractice insurance provides coverage if the policy was in effect when the incident took place, even if it is no longer in effect?**

   A. Claims-based insurance

   B. Occurrence-based insurance

   C. Malpractice tail insurance

   D. None

Answers: 1-D, 2-B

TASK 4: EMERGENCY PREPAREDNESS

An important part of any risk management plan is an emergency or crisis plan. Emergencies can result in several negative consequences, such as loss of revenue, injuries, anxiety, fear, and damage to property and important records. Being prepared for the most common types of emergencies your medical practice is likely to face can help to prevent or at least minimize these consequences.

Part of creating your practice's risk management plan is first conducting a hazard identification and vulnerability analysis. One way to accomplish this analysis is by using the Federal Emergency Management Agency (FEMA) recommendations and tools. According to FEMA, the risk management plan should:

- Identify hazards
- Profile hazard events
- Include a list of the organization's assets
- Estimate the potential human and economic losses, based on exposure and vulnerability

KEY TERM

Mitigation: The process of reducing the severity or impact of a negative event.

To identify potential hazards, practices should look at both external and internal conditions. External conditions include potential hazards associated with weather, such as tornadoes, hurricanes, lightning strikes, and flooding. Internal conditions that become hazardous include stairwells, chemical and pharmaceutical storage, biohazards storage, and similar elements. Not all of these conditions will apply to every practice.

Once you have identified the most likely hazards, analyze their potential of occurring (the frequency of such events in the past, for example, and the possibility of another occurrence), the practice's vulnerability to those hazards, and the potential losses involved. The practice should also look at vulnerability in terms of the most vulnerable places in the practice that could be damaged during an event. Then, create a plan that accounts for the most likely hazardous events and the most vulnerable assets.

The most common and probable hazards and events, according to OSHA,[18] are:

- Workplace violence
- Infectious disease
- Ergonomic issues
- Medical emergencies
- Hazardous chemicals
- Hazardous waste

- Natural disasters
- Loss of utilities
- Loss of electronic medical records
- Fires
- Other hazards and events

Workplace violence is a very real threat in our daily working lives. In 2016, workplace violence accounted for about 17% of on-the-job deaths, while the cost associated with those injuries was incalculable. According to the Bureau of Labor Statistics, homicides in the healthcare industry accounted for 4% of the total number of workplace homicides across all industries in 2018.[19]

Most attackers and harassers are people the victims deal with on a daily basis. Typical perpetrators of workplace violence are bitter, dissatisfied people who make threats of violence. Other types include:

- Frustrated employees who are shuffled from low-level tasks to even lower-level tasks
- Frustrated professionals
- Those who refuse to accept blame for their own problems
- Those with pent-up rage
- Those engaging in substance abuse
- Those experiencing extreme stress in their personal lives or with their jobs
- Those with little or no support systems, such as families or friends

Characteristics of at-risk work environments include group practices with:

- A strict authoritarian management style
- Numerous grievances filed
- Many disciplinary actions and/or terminations
- Inconsistent, inequitable, or insensitive management
- Chronic labor-management disputes
- Multiple injury claims
- Frequent layoffs and downsizing
- Disgruntled employees
- Interpersonal conflicts on the job
- Failure to recognize — and intervene — early in the cycle of violence

Ineffective or incompetent management contributes to workplace violence by failing to:

- Promptly respond to pre-employment warning signs or clues of future violence
- Admit that a potentially violent situation has occurred
- Follow-up after warning behaviors

- Communicate an expectation of self-control to the involved employee
- Convey that the employee will be held responsible for their inappropriate and unacceptable behavior

Workplace violence also affects employees' morale and productivity, increases absenteeism, promotes worker turnover, and raises costs for security and workers' compensation.

The World Health Organization and Centers for Disease Control provide guidelines for healthcare providers to follow to protect employees and patients from infection, infectious diseases, and exposure to epidemics. These guidelines can change depending on the type of epidemic or infection that is being controlled. Practices should have an infection control plan in place and guidelines for when it will be enacted. For example, during the COVID-19 pandemic, additional measures were needed to prevent the spread of the virus. These measures changed frequently as more was learned about how the virus spreads.

A designated person, such as the practice safety or compliance person, should stay informed of all recommended steps and guidelines for infection control and ensure the practice is meeting them. The person should also be in charge of communicating any new or changed standards and regulations to employees. Public health departments, as well as state and national public health organizations, require cases of some infectious diseases to be reported to them.

Medical emergencies can occur not just to patients visiting the healthcare facility, but also to employees and caregivers. An important part of a risk management plan is communicating with all employees to provide information about what to do in the event of a medical emergency of anyone at the practice. This plan should include the warning signs of emergencies, the first line of response (such as CPR), and how to contact the person's family in the event they are taken to the hospital. The plan should also include a specific policy and procedure about what to do during a medical crisis event, especially since each practice will have different equipment available for emergencies.

Figure 5.2[20]

Type of Office	Most Common Medical Emergencies*
Primary Care	Asthma exacerbation, Psychiatric, Seizure, Hypoglycemia, Anaphylaxis, Impaired consciousness, Shock, Poisoning, Drug overdose, Cardiac arrest
Child Care	Asthma exacerbation, Severe respiratory distress (non-asthma), Meningitis/sepsis, Seizure, Apnea, Anaphylaxis, Shock, Obstructed airway, Probable epiglottitis, Cardiac arrest
**Listed in order of frequency*	

Chemicals that are used throughout the workday, such as alcohol, disinfectants, and sterilant, are considered hazardous materials. Because of this, OSHA standard 29 CFR 1910.1200 discusses regulations and requirements for handling these chemicals. Its main requirements include:

- A written hazard communication program
- List of hazardous materials used or stored at the practice
- A safety data sheet (SDS) for each hazardous material on-site

OSHA lists six steps to providing an effective hazard communication program:

1. Learn the standard and identify staff responsible
2. Prepare and present the written communication program
3. Ensure containers are labeled
4. Maintain all SDS
5. Orient, inform, and train employees
6. Evaluate and reassess the program on a routine basis

Your practice can accomplish the first step by obtaining a copy of the Hazard Communication Standard. Next, the practice should assign an employee to be the primary person responsible for the program. This person can then identify other employees to perform activities related to the program, such as training. The written communication program needs to provide the details of how hazard communication will be handled by the practice. It also should provide a complete list of all the hazardous materials stored and used by the practice.

Medical practices also create hazardous waste products, such as bandages, syringes and sharps, and similar items. According to the U.S. Environmental Protection Agency (EPA), medical waste disposal is regulated at the state level since the 1988 Medical Waste Tracking Act expired in 1991. Your practice's safety department or person should be familiar with all hazardous waste disposal requirements at the state and local levels and ensure the practice meets them.[21]

Medical practices depend on utilities such as electricity and water to be able to function. Some emergencies, such as severe thunderstorms, flooding, tornadoes, earthquakes, and other natural disasters, may result in the loss of power and/or water to the facility. Like hospitals, medical practices should invest in generators that have capacity to meet the power needs of the building until power is restored. Emergency water and heating supplies or equipment should also be available, and employees trained to operate them. Equipment, supplies, and instructions should be part of the practice's emergency plan.

To avoid loss of medical records, practices should research and choose data backup systems. Data backup should occur regularly, using more than one system in case that system fails. Data storage servers should have reliable uninterrupted power supplies, and IT employees should know how to check backups and safely check all computer systems and servers.

The practice is also responsible for keeping patients' health records and personal information protected. The key factors to keep in mind when developing a system of ensuring EMR is available and not lost are:[22]

- Availability
- Having multiple systems
- Keeping records secure
- Accountability

OSHA requires all businesses, including medical practices, to comply with its standards (29 CFR Subpart E 1910.35, 1910.36, 1910.37, 1910.38, 1910.39) for exit routes and emergency plans. OSHA defines an exit route as a "continuous and unobstructed path of exit travel from any point within a workplace to a place of safety." The standard states that most buildings should have at least two exits. However, smaller facilities may meet the standard with one exit if all people in the building can exit from it safely. The OSHA standard states that exit routes must be permanent parts of the facility. Exit discharges (the part of the exit that leads directly outside) must be large enough to hold all of the people that will be exiting.

Other exit route requirements your practice should know include:

- Exits must be separated from the building by fire-resistant materials
- Exit route doors must be kept unlocked from the inside
- An exit access must be 28 inches wide at all points
- Exit routes must support the maximum number of occupants permitted in the building
- Exit routes must be kept unobstructed and a clear distance away from any hazardous or combustible materials
- Any doors along an exit route that are not exits should be clearly marked so people know they cannot use them as exits
- Exit doors should be clearly marked using the word EXIT
- Signs must be posted along the exit route notifying occupants of the way to the exit
- Lighting must illuminate the path and exit signs

Practices with more than 10 employees must also create and communicate a fire prevention plan. The minimum requirements of this plan are:

- List all major fire hazards
- Create procedures to control accumulation of flammable or combustible materials
- Ensure regular maintenance on all equipment that could accidentally ignite a fire
- Record and make available the name, title, and contact information of person responsible for maintaining equipment and fuel source hazards

Employees must also be notified when hired if there are any fire hazards they will be exposed to on the job.

Mitigation is the process of reducing the severity or impact of a negative event such as a natural disaster, fire, flood, violence in the workplace, and other issues discussed in this volume. A mitigation plan seeks to minimize the potential damages by putting structures, equipment, and plans in place to protect people, property, and data in the event of an emergency. The mitigation plan should be part of the risk management plan. The risk management team or person should look at what steps can be taken before the event to soften its impact. For example, practices located where tornadoes frequently occur may want to create a shelter in a lower level of the building where people could go during a tornado warning. The shelter could also be the place where important supplies are taken or stored, such as bottled water, a few days' supply of food, and emergency medical supplies.

Being prepared for emergencies means more than conducting fire drills and having fire extinguishers placed throughout the building (although these are important parts of being prepared for potential fire hazards). Being prepared means the organization has identified the most likely events that could occur, has determined what effects those events could have on people and the business, and has taken steps to mitigate the damage that could be the result of an occurrence. Keep in mind that emergencies generally fall into three categories: environmental/natural disasters, medical emergencies, and emergencies related to violence.

An emergency plan should address all three categories, and the risk management plan should also address them by considering the following aspects:

- Protocols and procedures
- Insurance
- Data backup and recovery
- Creating a continuity of operations plan (COOP)
- Employee training (providers and staff)
- Response equipment
- Response plan
- Recovery plan

For each category of emergency, and for each event listed in the plan, provide protocols and procedures for staff to follow. These can include calling 911, directing an evacuation plan, or ensuring employees know where to shelter during a tornado.

Data backup and recovery are vitally important to the medical practice, especially when patients' health records are electronic, and so are the practice's financial accounts. Having an appropriate plan for regularly backing up all data, and knowing how to recover data if it is lost, must be part of the risk management and emergency plans. Work with an IT professional, either within the practice or an outside vendor, to create a backup routine and recovery plan.

The emergency plan should also address how the practice can operate during most emergency situations. For example, when the practice loses electricity, a generator could be used. The practice should keep a supply of bottled water and other necessities on hand. The COOP should also include addressing how to operate with fewer employees in the event that public transportation is not available. During the COVID-19 pandemic, businesses were asked to keep numbers of employees to a minimum to prevent the spread of the virus. Making sure that employees are cross-trained and having a plan in place for operating with fewer staff members are important parts of an emergency plan.

Mitigation plans may include specific equipment in place to respond to certain emergencies. For example, fire extinguishers are required, and staff should be trained to use them. Data systems should have backup and storage equipment. Other equipment that may need to be in place includes generators, tools, flashlights, and protective equipment and gear.

The emergency plan should contain two separate sections for each type of emergency: an immediate response plan, and a recovery plan. The immediate response focuses on ensuring safety and security to the people on-site. All steps that need to be taken to immediately ensure the safety of those in the building make up the immediate response plan. Immediate response plans should also include how to notify staff members' emergency contacts, and police, fire, or other first responders as needed.

Disaster recovery planning is multi-faceted. Information technology functions are often the first area of planning to be reviewed.

However, the healthcare executive must review the entire business as part of the planning. If there is no access to the facility and the doctors cannot treat patients, there is no revenue. Without access to the bank, the practice is unable to process payroll or pay bills — or deposit additional funds. If there is no phone service, how do patients contact the practice for emergencies, appointments, or follow-up questions?

A disaster plan consists of precautions to be taken so that the impact of a disaster will be minimized, and the organization can resume critical functions. This planning can be divided into a six-stage cycle. The stages are risk assessment, business impact analysis, strategy and business contingency plan development, business continuity plan development, testing, and maintenance.

Being prepared for emergencies is important not only for the patients your practice serves, but also for all of the employees and visitors you might have at your practice on any given day. Emergency preparedness can save lives, prevent injuries, and protect property.

SAMPLE QUESTIONS

1. **What federal government agency provides emergency risk management information and tools?**

   A. OSHA

   B. CMS

   C. FEMA

   D. OCR

2. **The immediate response plan focuses on ensuring safety and security to:**

   A. The people on-site

   B. The neighborhood

   C. Equipment and devices

   D. Practice property

Answers: 1-C, 2-A

TASK 5: CYBERSECURITY

Cybersecurity is the protection of electronic data and computer systems from criminal or unauthorized uses. In the healthcare industry, it is especially important to protect patients' personal and health information. Most practices and providers maintain patient charts and data using electronic devices. This was an intentional move on the part of the healthcare industry, driven by U.S. governmental laws and regulations to facilitate sharing of information. Keeping data like this allows providers to share information with one another instantly when consultations need to occur. It also makes billing and submitting patient charges to insurance providers more efficient. However, it comes with many risks and security challenges that practices need to consider and address.

KEY TERMS

Cybersecurity: The protection of electronic data and computer systems from criminal or unauthorized uses.

Endpoint: Devices used by end users, such as laptops, tablets, and desktop computers.

Healthcare information is especially vulnerable to attack. This is because patient records can contain valuable information that allows attackers to steal patients' identities, get access to sensitive healthcare information, or gain access to payment and credit card information. Risks include security breaches that can occur when sending emails or submitting insurance claims. Improper use of devices by poorly trained staff can lead to exposed patient information, either accidentally or intentionally.

HIPAA's Privacy and Security Rules were issued to protect patient privacy and information. Privacy Rule standards specify how covered health information (protected health information, or PHI) can be used for treatment and billing of patients, as well as how it should be protected. HIPAA's goal is to protect health information while also ensuring information necessary for treating patients flows efficiently among providers and insurers.

The Security Rule states that confidential electronic protected health information, or e-PHI, cannot accidentally or intentionally be made available or disclosed to anyone who is not authorized to receive it. The Security Rule's confidentiality requirements go hand in hand with the Privacy Rule's stipulations about uses and disclosures of PHI; one does not conflict with the other.

The Security Rule describes the following administrative safeguards that all entities, including medical practices, must take in order to protect e-PHI:

- Managing security: As explained in the previous section, a practice must identify and analyze what its risks are when it comes to e-PHI and implement appropriate security measures that will reduce any identified risks and vulnerabilities.

- Designating personnel: Medical practices must designate an employee who is officially responsible for developing and implementing the security policies and procedures of the medical practice.
- Managing information access: Medical practices must decide what information is the minimum necessary e-PHI to maintain and communicate, and they must ensure policies and procedures are in place to support those minimum necessary guidelines. Practices should also ensure that the appropriate information is given to authorized requesters only.
- Training employees: Medical practices are required to develop appropriate levels of information access for all of their employees and then train and supervise employees as needed to ensure compliance with security policies and procedures. This also includes sanctions against employees who violate security and privacy policies and procedures.
- Evaluating security procedures: Medical practices are required under the Security Rule to assess their security procedures on a regular basis to ensure they meet all requirements and are effectively protecting e-PHI.

The Security Rule describes the following physical safeguards that all covered entities, including medical practices, must take in order to protect e-PHI:

- Controlling facility access: Medical practices need to define which employees will have access to secure facilities and physical access to records and equipment that contain e-PHI. They must also ensure that those who need the access have been given the authority required to do so.
- Securing workstations and devices: Medical practices are required to create and implement specific guidelines for how employees use and access workstations and other electronic media. Practices must also have policies in place that detail the proper transfer, removal, disposal, or reuse of electronic media. A covered entity must implement policies and procedures to specify proper use of and access to workstations and electronic media. A covered entity also must have in place policies and procedures regarding the transfer, removal, disposal, and reuse of electronic media, to ensure appropriate protection of e-PHI.

The Security Rule describes the following technical safeguards that all covered entities, including medical practices, must take in order to protect e-PHI:

- Controlling access: Access control refers to a practice's policies for ensuring that only authorized persons are able to access e-PHI. This may be the responsibility of the designated security person.
- Audit mechanisms: Under the Security Rule, practices must use hardware, software, or other mechanisms that record and examine how e-PHI is accessed and used by information systems that contain it.

- Controlling data integrity: Practices are expected to take steps to ensure that e-PHI is not altered or destroyed, whether intentionally or accidentally. Policies and procedures must dictate how to mitigate this kind of risk.
- Securing data transmission: Medical practices are required under the Security Rule to implement technical security measures that guard against unauthorized access to e-PHI that is being transmitted over an electronic network.

OCR can only act on complaints that meet the following criteria:

- The alleged incident took place when the rules were in effect
- The complaint is filed against an organization that is mandated to comply with the rules
- The complaint must describe an incident that is in violation of the rules
- The complaint must be filed within 180 days of the person finding out about the incident

In addition to third-party complaints, if an organization discovers a security breach in which health information was exposed, the organization must notify the Secretary of Health and Human Services. All notifications must be submitted using the web portal on the HHS website. An organization's breach notification obligations differ depending on whether the breach affected 500 or more people, or fewer than 500 people.

There are several types of breaches that can occur at any organization, but some of the more common ones are:

- Hacking/IT incident
- Improper disposal of paper records
- Loss of paper or electronic PHI
- Theft of mobile devices and/or paper records

Practices should keep in mind that breaches can occur anywhere and at any time, including:

- Desktop, laptop and tablet computers
- Email that is unencrypted
- Electronic Medical Record (EMR)
- Network servers
- Smart phone
- Paper files

Endpoints are the devices used by end users such as laptops, tablets, and desktop computers. They are at the "end" of the network. It is important to protect these devices for many reasons, including their vulnerability to attacks from hackers. If a hacker can access one employee laptop that is connected to the practice network, they may be able to hack into the network from there.

Also, more people are using their personal devices for work. This is called BYOD, or bring your own device. These personal devices also need to be protected when being used for work purposes.

Endpoint protection entails the following:[23]

- Network access control (administration of passwords)
- Examining files as they enter the network
- Malware (computer software with malicious intent) detection
- Application controls
- Encryption of data

Networks are also usually connected to the internet and are therefore vulnerable to attack. To protect the network, there are both hardware and software solutions available. These include:[24]

- Firewalls (hardware, software, or both): Use a set of rules to allow or block incoming and outgoing "traffic"
- Email security: Blocks incoming email attacks and controls outbound messages that may contain sensitive data (see below for more information)
- Antivirus and anti-malware software
- Access control helps the practice recognize users and devices so no unauthorized user or device can access the network
- Application security ensures all software applications used by the practice are protected and secure
- Web security blocks web-based threats and access to malicious websites

Users should be trained to identify suspicious emails they may receive. Called phishing, emails can appear to be from trusted sources such as banking or insurance institutions. Usually, they notify people that their account needs to be verified or a similar request. To verify the account, the user is supposed to click on a link. Users should be trained to scrutinize the email address of the sender, and to hover their mouse or cursor over any link to see the URL address. If it is not directly to the organization the email claims to be from, it is an attempt to gain identifying information from the user, and the message should be deleted or forwarded to an IT advisor for further scrutiny. Users should be advised never to open attachments in suspicious-looking emails, and to report all phishing attempts to the IT person or department.

All practices' email systems should be encrypted for protection and to meet HIPAA privacy regulations when exchanging patient information. All email protection systems should be updated regularly.

Network executives should ensure that access to networks is secure and that when an employee joins or leaves the practice their access changes accordingly. Executives can also keep the network secure by ensuring that employees only have access to the network functions and computer applications that are needed to perform their work. Access to patient information should be restricted to those who need it to perform their jobs.

Cybersecurity policies and procedures will differ from practice to practice, depending on the size of the practice, how many facilities it has, and how many and what types of devices are being used. Each practice should create policies and procedures that ensure that cybersecurity measures are in place, in use, employees understand them, and that they meet all applicable laws and regulations, including HIPAA laws.

Computer systems and networks are under constant and changing threats, and the IT department should keep up to date on the most recent attacks. The practice may need to modify protection systems. Policies and procedures should be documented thoroughly and be available for all employees to refer to. When updates occur, all employees should be informed.

Backup refers to a system in which data is copied to a storage device on a regular basis. Recovery provides access to that stored data. This is critical in case the data is lost for any reason. A backup system allows the data to be restored quickly and easily. Backup systems may be located on-site and off-site or on a cloud device, which is a server that doesn't belong to the practice, stores data for multiple people or businesses, and can be accessed via the internet. Since cloud backup systems are operated by people outside the practice, they should be chosen wisely and only reputable, well-known companies that can assure appropriate encryption of data should be considered.

Keep in mind that not all data should be backed up or can be retrieved. For some very critical data, hard paper copies may be important to have and kept in secure filing systems.

New technologies for cybersecurity can add extra protection or sharpen the focus of your practice's current protection systems. A few of these include:[25]

- Predictive analytics (analyzes security data and predicts possible areas of attack)
- Machine learning (uses algorithms to create models and predictions)
- Behavioral analytics (detects patterns in network and system activity)

Many of today's medical devices are computerized and typically connect to a practice's network via the internet for ease of recording and sharing information. However, that also makes them vulnerable to attacks. Recognizing this, the Medical Imaging & Technology Alliance (MITA) released a medical device security standard that includes advice for healthcare providers to use to ensure their devices are secure. The standards also recommend that manufacturers work with providers to create and implement controls. The standard, Manufacturer Disclosure Statement for Medical Device Security (MDS2), works in conjunction with the U.S. Food and Drug Administration Medical Device Cybersecurity Playbook. Practices should be familiar with the standard and guidance, and can become familiar by visiting the FDA website.[26]

Practices should conduct yearly assessments to determine whether their cybersecurity measures meet regulations and are effective in keeping data secure. If your practice has not conducted an assessment before and is unsure of how to do one, the Office of Homeland Security offers guidelines at its website on a range of assessments companies can perform. The practice should select an assessment method that will work best for it and that includes examining endpoint security, network security, and medical device security.[27]

Assessments can be performed inhouse by the practice's network or IT staff members. Other members of the practice, including those who provide patient care, should also be part of the team, so that knowledge of how all devices are used is accurate and up to date. The practice can hire an outside firm to complete an assessment. This can also lead to more objective or reliable results. Practices should carefully choose the company to perform the assessment, as well as have clear, set goals for it.

The Federal Communications Commission also provides a Cybersecurity Planning Guide businesses may use as part of their assessment or audit system and/or to help develop a plan for cybersecurity.[28]

Once the cybersecurity assessment has been completed and any necessary upgrades, updates, and changes have been made to improve security, the team should also complete a review of the practice's cybersecurity policies. Revisions to these policies should reflect any changes made to the practice's cybersecurity practices as a result of the assessment. All agreements should also be updated, including any signed agreements by users to abide by the practice's cybersecurity and computer use policies.

If the practice feels it is especially vulnerable in any one aspect of cybersecurity, using one of these assessment tools may be an important prevention strategy. Penetration tests are conducted to test the security of a network. They should be performed periodically to ensure that a network's security measures are working. This is also called ethical hacking. Usually, outside companies or individuals certified to perform these tests will conduct them so the practice is assured that its data will not be in danger if security measures are breached.

In addition to cybersecurity tools and assessments, practices may want to consider purchasing cybersecurity insurance.[29] This insurance protects practices from the effects of a data breach or hack in which sensitive information is released. In the event that protected personal or health information, as well as insurance and credit card information is accessed, it can be very costly to recover. Following a large data breach, there is the possibility of legal suits, as well as the cost of reimbursing patients in the event of unauthorized charges on their credit cards. As with any other type of insurance, practices should assess the likelihood of a large breach, the costs the practice might incur if one occurs, and whether the protection offered by insurance is worth the cost of the insurance premiums.

It is not enough to conduct assessments and testing. It is important that medical practices develop a plan that includes preparing for:

- Privacy and data security
- Scams and fraud
- Network security
- Website security
- Email

- Mobile devices
- Facility and operational security
- Staff security
- Patient security

Helpful resources include the FCC's Cybersecurity Planning Guide.

Employees need to be aware that threats may occur at any time. Employees should learn the warning signs that their personal devices, computers, or email accounts have been breached. These signs include:

- New applications on the computer
- Browser activity not recognized by the user
- Odd emails and email addresses appearing in email account
- Passwords will not work

If your practice does not have a dedicated team of employees to handle IT matters, or lacks expertise in cybersecurity, the practice should consider hiring a company to provide these services. If finding time to train employees becomes challenging, consider developing an online training system employees can use at their own convenience, or offering the training after hours.

SAMPLE QUESTIONS

1. **The HIPAA Security Rule states that a designated person at the practice is responsible for:**

   A. Developing and implementing the IT security policies and procedures of the medical practice

   B. Hiring and firing security staff members of the medical practice

   C. Developing and implementing risk management policies and procedures of the medical practice

   D. Developing and implementing the security policies and procedures of the medical practice

2. **All practice email systems should be _______ for protection.**

   A. encrypted

   B. shut down daily

   C. monitored

   D. cleaned out

Answers: 1-D, 2-A

RISK AND COMPLIANCE MANAGEMENT QUIZ

1. **What type of insurance does a practice need to purchase to protect its physical assets?**

   A. Unemployment

   B. Malpractice

   C. Property and casualty

   D. Employment liability

2. **The Health Insurance Portability and Accountability Act pertains to:**

   A. Billing insurance companies' compliance rules

   B. Obtaining insurance after employment ends

   C. Standards for privacy of identifiable health information

   D. Occupational health and safety

3. **Which three categories do most emergencies fall under?**

   A. Infectious disease, ergonomic issues, and hazardous chemicals

   B. Hazardous waste, loss of utilities, and loss of electronic medical records

   C. Environmental/natural disasters, medical emergencies, and emergencies related to violence

   D. Fires, hazardous chemicals, and loss of utilities

4. **________ is the process of reducing the severity or impact of a negative event.**

   A. Insurance

   B. Risk assessment

   C. Compliance

   D. Mitigation

ANSWERS

1-B. Malpractice insurance does not protect a practice's physical assets.

2-C. HIPAA provides standards and guidelines for keeping health information private.

3-C. Most emergencies that occur in medical practices fall into three categories: environmental/natural disasters, medical emergencies, and emergencies related to violence.

4-D. Mitigation is the process of reducing the severity or impact of a negative event.

Notes

1. G.L. Head and S. Horn, *Essentials of Risk Management*, vol. 1 (Malvern, PA: Insurance Institute of America, 1991), 6.
2. J. Reason, *Human Error* (Cambridge, UK: Cambridge University Press, 1990), 208.
3. R.E. McDermott, R.J. Mikulak, and M.R. Beauregard, *The Basics of FMEA* (Portland, OR: Productivity, 1996), 1-5.
4. Head and Horn, *Essentials*, vol. 1, 8.
5. G.L. Head and S. Horn, *Essentials of Risk Management*, vol. 2 (Malvern, PA: Insurance Institute of America, 1991), 13.
6. Ibid, 40.
7. Ibid, 162.
8. L.T. Kohn, J.M. Corrigan, M.S. Donaldson. *To Err is Human: Building a Safer Health System* (Washington, DC: National Academy Press, Institute of Medicine, 1999).
9. Gary Bennett, "Managing Risk for Clients and for Ourselves. A Bug's Life (and the Turnbull Report)," *Risk Management at PB: Balancing Risk and Reward* 16, no. 51 (January 2002): 3.
10. U.S. Department of Health and Human Services, Office of Inspector General (HHS/OIG), OIG Compliance Program for Individual and Small Group Physician Practices , 65 Fed. Reg. 194, Oct. 5, 2000, p. 1, https://oig.hhs.gov/authorities /docs/ physician.pdf.
11. Occupational Safety and Health Administration, *Hazard Communication: Small Entity Compliance Guide for Employers That Use Hazard Chemicals* (OSHA, U.S. Department of Labor 3695-03, 2014), www.osha.gov /Publications/OSHA3695.pdf.
12. U.S. Department of Health and Human Services, Office of Inspector General (HHS/OIG) *Medicare Program: Reporting and Returning of Overpayments*, 81 Fed. Reg. 29, Feb. 12, 2016, https://www.govinfo.gov/content/pkg/FR-2016-02-12/pdf/2016-02789.pdf.
13. U.S. Department of Health and Human Services, Office of Inspector General (HHS/OIG) *Compliance Program Guidance for Hospitals*, 63 Fed. Reg. 8987, Feb. 23, 1998, p. 4, https://oig.hhs.gov/authorities/docs /cpghosp.pdf.
14. *A Roadmap for New Physicians: Avoiding Medicare and Medicaid Fraud and Abuse, Physician Education Training Materials*, U.S. Department of Health and Human Services, Office of Inspector General, https://oig.hhs.gov/compliance/physician-education/index.asp.
15. Medical Group Management Association, "Credentialing Process." All rights reserved.

16. American College of Physicians, "Medical Malpractice Insurance," Residency Career Guidance, https://www.acponline.org/about-acp/about-internal-medicine/career-path.
17. Scott Dutton, "What is Malpractice Tail Coverage?" The Student Doctor Network, November 28, 2012.
18. "Other Hazards," Safety and Health Topics, U.S. Department of Labor, Occupational Safety and Health Administration, osha.gov/SLTC/healthcarefacilities/otherhazards.html.
19. "Fact Sheet Workplace Violence in Healthcare, 2018," U.S. Department of Labor, Bureau of Labor Statistics, bls.gov/iif/oshwc/cfoi/work_violence-healthcare-2018.
20. C.L. Johnston, M.G. Coulthard, P.J. Schluter, M.L. Dick. "Medical emergencies in general practice in south-east Queensland: prevalence and practice preparedness," Med J Aust. 2001;175:99-103; American Academy of Pediatrics, Division of Child Health Research. Periodic Survey No. 27. Emergency readiness of pediatric offices. Elk Grove Village, Ill.: American Academy of Pediatrics, 1995.
21. "Medical Waste," United States Environmental Protection Agency, epa.gov/rcra/medical-waste.
22. T. Eric Schackow, Todd Palmer, Ted Epperly, "HER Meltdown: How to Protect Your Patient Data," American Academy of Family Physicians, June 2008.
23. Nate Lord, "What is Endpoint Protection? Data Protection 101." Data Insider, Digital Guardian, September 10, 2018.
24. "What is Network Security?" Cisco, Cisco.com.
25. Steve Alder, "MTA Publishes New Medical Device Security Standard," HIPAA Journal, October 14, 2019.
26. "Cybersecurity," U.S. Food & Drug Administration, Digital Health, Medical Devices, March 3, 2020.
27. "Risk and Vulnerability Assessment," Cyber Resource Hub, Department of Homeland Security, Last revised May 29, 2020.
28. "Cyber Security Planning Guide," Federal Communications Commission, https://transition.fcc.gov/cyber/cyberplanner.pdf.
29. "What is Cybersecurity Insurance?" CyberInsure One, Cyber Insurance FAQ, https://cyberinsureone.com/faq/what-is-cyber-security-insurance.

Chapter 6

Organizational Governance

Business executives in all industries are responsible for providing broad organizational leadership and for defining and achieving corporate goals. Healthcare executives are no exception.

This section provides a blueprint designed by practicing healthcare executives to describe the key competencies, knowledge, and skills required to organize and govern the medical practice.

The major areas of competence in organizational governance, as identified by the certified and Fellowed members of the Medical Group Management Association (MGMA), are:

1. Corporate Mission, Vision, and Values
2. Legal Structure and Governance
3. Organizational Policy and Procedures

TASK 1: CORPORATE MISSION, VISION, AND VALUES

The quality of an organization's culture is a key determinant of its success or failure. A strong, positive culture can lead to a medical practice's success, while a dysfunctional or undefined culture can make it difficult or impossible for the practice to achieve its goals.

Culture is the foundation of corporate identity. Culture reflects the practice's most closely held values and beliefs, guides day-to-day decision-making, and governs how decisions are implemented.

When trying to implement new strategies or a strategic plan, healthcare executives will often discover that their strategies will fail if they are implementing programs that are inconsistent with the organization's culture.

KEY TERMS

Organizational culture: An organization's self-sustaining patterns of behaving, feeling, thinking and believing.

Mission statement: Explains why an organization exists, describes the services it provides, who its customers are, and how services will be delivered.

Values statement: Defines the organization's most deeply held beliefs, which form the foundation of its corporate identity.

Vision statement: Defines the organization's aspirations for the future.

1.1 Organizational Culture

One widely accepted definition of culture is "the way things are done around here."[1] Peter Drucker, renowned management theorist and educator, expanded this definition when he wrote that "Culture is an organization's self-sustaining patterns of behaving, feeling, thinking and believing."[2] Drucker's definition shows that culture can determine an organization's self-image, its external image, and the way it operates. In other words, just about everything related to an organization is defined by its culture.

Drucker emphasized the centrality of culture when he wrote that "Culture eats strategy for breakfast." Drucker's comment implies that the best business plans and strategies will fail if they are not supported by a robust and enthusiastic culture.

In his book, *Organizational Culture and Leadership*,[3] Edward Schein presents five guidelines for understanding corporate culture:

1. Do not oversimplify culture or confuse it with climate, values, or corporate philosophy. Culture underlies, supports, and largely determines these other factors of an organization.
2. Do not label culture as solely a human resource aspect of an organization, affecting only its human side.
3. Do not assume that practice leadership can manipulate culture in the same way leaders might seek to control other aspects of the organization.
4. Do not assume there is a "right" or "wrong" culture, or that one type of culture is necessarily superior to another.
5. Do not assume that all the aspects of organizational culture are important or will have a major effect on how it functions.

McKinsey and Company[4] defined four reasons that corporate culture matters:

1. Culture correlates with performance
2. Culture is unique to every organization, cannot be readily duplicated by competitors, and is essential for the practice to differentiate itself in the market
3. Organizations that have performance-driven cultures adapt more successfully to environmental changes and enjoy a competitive advantage over organizations that are resistant to change
4. Unhealthy cultures can lead to underperformance or worse

Identifying and transforming a practice's corporate culture requires advanced skills on the part of the healthcare executive that can only be developed with time and experience.

The components essential for building a corporate culture are mission, vision, and values. Another important component for healthcare practices is the commitment to creating a high-reliability and zero-harm organization. In combination, all of these components can create a highly productive culture that motivates and rewards employees to meet corporate goals while delivering the highest possible levels of safety and quality patient care.

An important cultural component that sometimes can be overlooked is the organization's need to understand and be continually in compliance with all federal and state regulations. While sometimes seen as bothersome in the healthcare industry, these regulatory requirements are designed to encourage the delivery of only medically necessary patient care in a financially and legally responsible way.

The governing body and healthcare executive are responsible for creating, implementing, and maintaining a compliance-driven culture, and for ensuring that this culture is understood and adopted throughout the medical practice.

Developing and personally communicating the organization's corporate mission, vision, and values statements are critical responsibilities for the healthcare executive and should never be delegated to someone who has a lower-level role in leadership. Staff buy-in of the corporate mission, vision, and values statements may be predicated on their belief that the healthcare executive helped to develop, fully understands, and completely supports them.[5]

Figure 6.1[6]

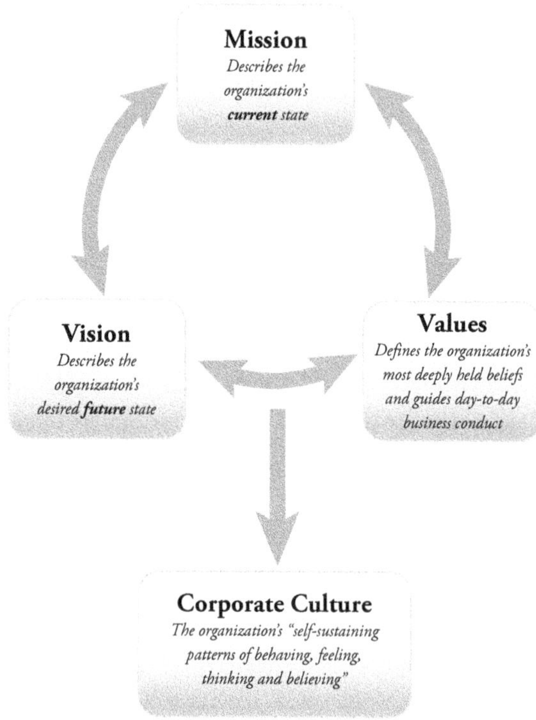

The mission statement explains why an organization exists, describes the services it provides, who its customers are, and how services will be delivered. From a leadership perspective, an effective mission statement:

- Outlines the organization's approach for fulfilling its purpose
- Creates staff loyalty and motivates them by explaining the organization's purpose and demonstrating the leadership's commitment to fulfilling it
- Provides healthcare executives with a way to measure whether the organization is moving closer to or further from its goals

The most effective corporate mission statements are:

- Succinct and sufficiently brief to be printed on the back of a business card.
- Memorable and easy for practice staff to remember and recite.
- Plainly written and easy to understand (an overly long or complex statement can limit understanding and reduce organization-wide buy-in).
- Organization-specific; describes the practice's purpose in a unique and non-generic way.
- Realistic and credible. The mission statement is not an aspirational document; its purpose is to define why the organization exists, the services it provides, and who it serves.

It is important to include input from stakeholders at all organizational levels, including the governing body (board of directors), providers, the executive leadership team, managers, and staff. Broad-based stakeholder participation in the development process improves the quality, organizational understanding, and buy-in of the corporate mission statement.

Practices that recognize changes in their environment, and effectively adjust to those changes, have a significant competitive advantage over those that do not. Skillful change management can make the difference between successful group practices and those that are left behind.

The vision statement is forward-facing and optimistic by design, and should foster employee commitment by painting a picture of what the organization wants to accomplish in the future.

An effective vision statement also builds staff confidence in the organization by showing that the corporate mission will remain in place as the organization moves into the future. Basing the vision statement on the organization's mission lets staff know that no matter what the future holds, the organization will remain true to its purpose as it pursues its vision.

Best medical practice vision statements are:

1. Future-oriented. The vision statement is not what the company is doing today, but rather sets a future objective or goal for where the company hopes to go.
2. Concise. The vision statement should be simple and easy to read so that it can be easily remembered and repeated accurately.
3. Reflective of a company's culture and core values.
4. Optimistic, inspirational, and able to paint a bright picture of the future that rallies all staff members and employees to work toward a common goal.
5. Challenging. Corporate vision is aspirational and should take a bold view when setting future goals.
6. Realistic, attainable, and seen as credible to leadership and staff. While the vision should not be too easy to achieve, it also should not be so unrealistic that employees feel it will be impossible to achieve, and so ignore it.
7. Clear. A good rule of thumb for clarity is to focus on one primary goal, rather than trying to fill the document with several scattered ideas. One clear objective is also easier to focus on and achieve.
8. Tied to the corporate mission and shows that the practice's purpose will remain unchanged as the organization moves into the future.
9. Stable. The vision statement should neither be driven by market forces or developments, nor require changes in the organization's corporate mission.
10. General in nature. The vision statement should be broad enough to capture the organization's overall interests and future direction. To be

credible, the vision statement should define organizational aspirations for the near- to mid-term.

A corporate values statement defines the organization's most deeply held beliefs which form the foundation of its corporate identity. While the corporate mission defines what the organization is and its purpose, values represent how the organization will endeavor to achieve that mission on a daily basis.

Effective values statements are:

1. Unique to each organization and reflect how employees think and feel about the organization at the moment.
2. Central to developing a high-performance culture. It is impossible to develop a high performing culture without values that define and support that behavior.
3. Collaborative in nature and should include input from staff at all levels of the organization.
4. More discovered than created. In other words, while corporate values can and should be deliberately defined, they ultimately depend more on how employees understand and practice them on a daily basis.
5. Not just a behavior but also a mindset.

Influencing corporate values is challenging, time-consuming, and requires healthcare executives to lead by example, consistently modeling the behaviors they desire in others at the practice every day. Practice staff members will not change their behavior until they see evidence that practice leaders believe the corporate values they espouse and are completely committed to putting them in place.

An important component of corporate culture, and one that should be explicitly reflected in the mission statement, is the practice's commitment to creating a "high-reliability" and "zero-harm" organization.

A high-reliability organization is supported by a culture of "collective mindfulness where workers look for, report, and address small problems or unsafe conditions when they are easy to fix, and long before they pose a major hazard."[7]

High-reliability cultures also encourage staff to do the analysis, critical thinking, and performance reporting required to continuously improve patient care systems, processes, and outcomes.

Establishing a high-reliability organization requires healthcare executive and board commitment to make patient safety the organization's number one goal. This also ensures that high reliability is reflected in the organization's culture. The organization is seen as valuing open and honest communication about ways to improve patient care systems and outcomes.

Practices should also aim to become zero-harm organizations. Even though no group practice can deliver perfect, completely error-free care, striving to achieve zero harm is an aspirational goal that should be an important component of culture. The commitment to becoming a zero-harm organization demonstrates the practice's dedication to continuously providing the highest possible levels of safe and quality patient care.

Robert E. Quinn and Kim S. Cameron of the University of Michigan[8] categorize corporate culture into four types: adhocracy, clan, hierarchy, and market.

Adhocracy culture is externally focused, adept at recognizing and adapting to change, and is characterized by high levels of innovation, experimentation, disruption, and risk-taking. This cultural type is most often seen in fast-paced, entrepreneurial organizations that demand a high level of flexibility in responding to market changes. It is common among tech companies that must strive to stay ahead of the competition when it comes to new products. In general, the adhocracy culture is usually appropriate or commonly used in medical practices.

Clan culture relies on personal relationships, collaboration, team building, employee engagement, human resources training and development, mentoring, and coaching to achieve its goals. This cultural type is most often seen in "high touch," people-oriented organizations where human resources are the most important asset. Most medical group practices' cultures are clan-oriented.

Hierarchy cultures emphasize efficiency, standardized processes, tight cost control, continual performance improvement, high levels of technical expertise, and advanced problem-solving. This cultural type is often seen in highly structured, bureaucratic organizations that must produce consistently high-quality products and outcomes to compete in a competitive market. Many medical practice cultures incorporate aspects of the hierarchy culture.

Market cultures are hard-driving and focused on delivering high shareholder value, competing for capital and market share, fast decision-making, and the consistent delivery of on-time results. Market cultures break down barriers and have directive and commanding leadership styles. This culture is best suited for a marketing- and sales-oriented organization responsible for getting products and services to market. Many medical practice cultures include elements of a market culture when they are provider-owned and focused on increasing and delivering shareholder value.

Larger, more complex practices (e.g., those that are structured as S or C corporations) that offer a broader range of services typically have cultures that incorporate elements of multiple culture types, including adhocracy, clan, and hierarchy. While these organizations may have an overarching culture, subsets of other culture types can develop in departments that are functionally distinct and require varying levels of expertise and problem-solving.

Smaller, less complex practices (e.g., sole proprietorships, or smaller professional associations or corporations) typically rely on the clan type of culture. In this type of culture, the quality of relationships and degree of collaboration among team members will determine the organization's success.

The coexistence of both of these cultural types in one organization, especially at the leadership level, can generate internal conflict as leaders try to balance the drive for increased profitability with the need to provide high quality care as efficiently as possible. Well-defined and accepted corporate values can aid in the reconciliation of these types of internal conflicts.

Practices that are owned by the providers as shareholders develop a culture based on the owners' priorities, goals, and values. Owners focused on improving shareholder value through increased profitability tend to be more risk tolerant and control-oriented. They foster cultures closely tied to the hierarchy and market types.

Shareholder-owned practices with a greater focus on internal and external relationships and the provision of patient care tend to be more risk averse and rely more heavily on the clan culture type. They may also include elements of the hierarchy type.

Practices that have a more corporate structure tend to have a relatively low risk tolerance, depend on well-defined management structures and tight process controls, and develop cultures most closely tied to the hierarchy and market types.

Practices owned by or affiliated with external provider-based or corporate entities tend to be risk averse, dependent on external leadership and management, have limited control over provider income, and share practice net profit with the "parent" organization. These organizations are often required to adopt at least some elements of the larger organization's culture and tend to develop a hierarchy culture to ensure that internal operations meet external corporate goals. They may also adopt the elements of a clan culture that are needed to successfully manage relationships with external owners.

A healthy culture is essential for any highly functioning medical practice. These cultures require thoughtfully developed statements of corporate mission, vision, and values. Defining and communicating the organization's corporate mission, vision, and values are critical to the success of the organization, and an important responsibility of the healthcare executive.

SAMPLE QUESTIONS

1. **What is the difference between an organization's mission and its values?**

   A. The corporate mission defines what the organization is and its purpose, while values represent how the organization will endeavor to achieve that mission on a daily basis

   B. The corporate mission paints a picture of what the organization wants to accomplish in the future, while values represent how the organization will endeavor to achieve that mission on a daily basis

   C. The corporate mission defines what the organization is and its purpose, while values paint a picture of what the organization wants to accomplish in the future

   D. The corporate mission defines the organization's vision, while values represent the organization's mission on a daily basis

2. **Which type of culture is adept at recognizing and adapting to change?**

   A. Adhocracy

   B. Clan

   C. Hierarchy

   D. Market

Answers: 1-A, 2-A

TASK 2: ORGANIZATION'S LEGAL STRUCTURE AND GOVERNANCE

Understanding the possible business structures available to medical practices and selecting the one that is most appropriate are essential skills for healthcare executives. Each business structure has specific legal, risk, and tax implications that can either serve the practice's needs or compromise them. Medical practice governing bodies and leaders often do not understand the features and potential impacts of different legal models, nor do they recognize how each may or may not advance corporate goals. A skilled healthcare executive must understand the types of business structures available, as well as the advantages and disadvantages of each one. Healthcare executives must be able to explain these structures to board members and other senior practice leaders. Choosing the best model depends on the legal risks and tax profile that best fit the practice's mission and goals.

KEY TERMS

Sole proprietorship: Organization with a single owner that is not established as a separate legal entity.

Professional corporation (PC): A distinct legal entity that exists separate from its owners.

Professional limited liability company (PLLC): Organizational structure that allows the profits from the limited liability partnership (LLP) to be taxed as partnerships.

Professional limited liability partnership (PLLP): Organizational structure that allows the profits from the limited liability company (LLC) to be taxed as partnerships.

2.1 Implications of the Legal Structure

The medical practice's business structure determines the tax liability exposure, the degree of flexibility in fulfilling corporate strategy, and helps to define physician compensation options. Therefore, the board and the healthcare executive should carefully define practice expectations in all of these areas.

Defining the practice's liability tolerance might appear straightforward. All practices want the lowest possible level of risk. However, this decision is more nuanced than it may appear, because while certain legal models provide extensive risk protection, they also can narrow the options practices will have for growing and responding to changes in their markets. For example, there are important differences across S corporations, C corporations, and limited liability partnerships and corporations (LLCs) that specify how taxes, net income, and retained earnings are recorded, and how or whether the income and earnings may be distributed as physician compensation. In addition, certain legal structures can simplify the acquisition of assets for growth, increase access to capital, and maximize practice value if the practice is considering being sold to or acquired by another company.

While the healthcare executive is responsible for recommending to the board the business structure that is the best fit, this process can be complex and require specialized legal and tax expertise unavailable within the organization. Outside expert advice is often worth the cost, because it is less expensive to choose the right legal model today than to correct an inappropriate choice in the future.

Most medical groups in the United States use one of the following models for establishing their business structure:

- Sole proprietorship
- Professional corporation (PC) or professional association (PA)
- Professional limited liability partnership (PLLP)
- Professional limited liability company (PLLC)

Few medical practices use either the general or limited partnership form of legal structure, mostly because these legal structures do not provide sufficient liability protection and can create significant tax disadvantages compared with other models. From a tax perspective, the Federal Internal Revenue Code and statutes define the tax implications of each business structure.

The most common business structures are sole proprietorships, professional and business corporations, professional limited liability partnerships, and professional limited liability companies.

A medical practice with a single physician owner that is not established as a separate legal entity is considered a sole proprietorship. In this structure, the assets of the individual physician and the medical practice are not separate, so the physician is not protected from any liability resulting from practice activities as they would be in a PC or similar structure. In other words, if the practice is unable to pay all of its debts and declares bankruptcy, the physician's personal funds would be included in the assets.

It is important to note that a solo practice is not the same thing legally as a sole proprietorship. A sole proprietorship is a formal legal structure, while a solo practice is not. A solo practice may be organized as a sole proprietorship, a PC, or similar legal structure that is owned by a single physician. Under these business structures, the physician can work in a solo practice format while receiving the liability protection of a corporation.

The advantages of a sole proprietorship include:

- Control: The physician-owner has total control over money and decisions because there are no partners or shareholders
- Flexibility: A sole proprietorship is relatively easy to set up and requires no separate tax filing

The disadvantages of a sole proprietorship include:

- There is no history for lending purposes. It can be difficult for a new medical practice to borrow funds without collateral or a history of borrowing.

- Backup may not be available. Another provider may not be readily available to provide coverage when the physician is unavailable.
- There is no liability protection. Because a sole proprietorship is not a separate legal entity, the owner is personally responsible for all practice liabilities.
- The sole proprietor has full responsibility for practice management. In addition to providing patient care, the owner is responsible for all of the practice's financial and operational decision.

Some practices choose to operate as a nonprofit organization or a nonprofit department in a larger organization. Nonprofit organizations are given 501(c)(3) tax status. Nonprofit organizations, by definition, are not legally permitted to accumulate profits. Instead, they are required to reinvest any profits they earn into the organization, facilities, or mission.

The advantages of being a nonprofit organization include:

- Exemption from paying income taxes
- Exemption from paying property taxes
- Other tax advantages can vary from state to state

The disadvantages of being a nonprofit organization include:

- Reliance on donors or on grants for funding
- Potential reliance on local community for support and funding
- Limitations on amount of funds that can be invested in financial vehicles before nonprofit status is compromised

A professional corporation (PC) is a distinct legal entity that exists separate from its owners. These types of organizations have four characteristics:

1. Limited liability
2. Continuity of existence
3. Transferability of ownership
4. Centralized management

A PC is a legal entity separate from its owners for liability protection and tax advantage purposes. A PC is generally subject to the same basic requirements and rules as any other business corporation, except that only licensed professionals may own or share an interest in it. Non-providers can neither own nor invest in a PC. In addition, PC ownership can be transferred only to another licensed professional.

A business corporation is also a separate legal entity that limits the liability of its owners. Unlike a PC, however, a business corporation allows outside investors as well as ownership by non-physicians.

While this legal structure shares most of the benefits of a PC (except taxation), this model is seldom used for medical practices because licensing laws in many states restrict medical practice ownership to licensed physicians.

The advantages of a corporate legal structure include:

- Limited liability. Shareholders are not responsible for corporate debt or practice-related liabilities.
- Additional tax deductions. Because the corporation pays employee and provider benefits, such as health and life insurance, those costs are tax deductible corporate expenses.
- Transferability. Ownership can be sold or transferred to another medically licensed person or entity.

The disadvantages of corporations include:

- Shareholders are double-taxed, first on corporate net income and again on personal income. Many practices can avoid this by organizing as an S corporation.
- Corporations require more complex governance and management structures with detailed reporting and documentation obligations.
- Corporations are required to have formal governance boards and typically also have very structured management models.

PLLPs and PLLCs provide different levels of legal protection or limited liability to the organization's owners. Both structures allow the profits from the limited liability partnership (LLP) or limited liability company (LLC) to be taxed as partnerships. This means there is no potential for double taxation of entity profits, as in the case of the C corporation model.

The procedure for setting up these or other forms of organizations is defined by state law, although most require the filing of articles of organization or similar shareholder documents.

Advantages of LLCs and LLPs:

- Limited personal liability. Shareholders are not responsible for corporate debt or practice-related liabilities.
- The medical practice is treated as a partnership for tax purposes, so income and losses are passed directly to the owners and are not subject to double taxation.

Disadvantages of LLCs and LLPs are:

- More complex governance.
- Physicians are not employees. Physicians generally are not employees of PLLPs or PLLCs, rendering them ineligible for benefits available in a PC or similar structure.
- Different financial management. Both entities require financial management practices somewhat different from those found in the more common PC form.
- Variable state laws. Not every state allows medical practices to use a PLLP or PLLC model.

2.2 Organizational Management Structure

Most organizations, including medical practices, are open systems. This means that operations are impacted by environmental factors, including government regulations, as well as social and market changes.

All of these can have a direct impact on how a medical practice operates, as well as the cost of operations. For example, when HIPAA was first enacted, healthcare providers had to make several changes to the way they operated, from providing written notices and posting signs advising patients of their right to privacy, to training employees about all of the HIPAA regulations. A practice's organizational governance can be impacted by these forces as well. For example, practices had to designate staff members to ensure HIPAA compliance, and leaders were responsible for ensuring oversight.

Organizational governance also must be community-focused when it comes to strategic management. Medical practices exist to meet the healthcare needs of the community, and each community has its own unique needs. Healthcare executives must keep those needs in mind when structuring governance of the practice.

Continuous improvement may also impact how a practice is governed and structured. As the practice engages in continuous improvement, changes may be needed in who makes decisions, for example. Continuous improvement may also lead to streamlining processes and removing some hierarchies of leadership.

Another environmental factor that impacts how a practice is governed is the scale of both the healthcare needs of the community, and the scale of the practice itself. Smaller practices or those focused on specialized care may require fewer managers, while large-scale operations may require more in order to meet patient and employee needs.

Customer or patient motivation may also impact practice strategies. If patients are highly motivated it means they usually participate more in their care and may ask for or require additional services. This may mean the practice needs additional providers or managers. Board member motivation will also impact governance. Board member focus and priorities will have a direct impact on how the practice is governed.

Most healthcare organizations, both large and small, seek to establish a governing board whose purpose is to ensure the organization has the tools and support necessary to carry out its mission. The governing board also provides oversight to ensure the practice or organization is providing quality medical care and meeting its goals.

The governing board also serves these functions:

- Appoints the chief executive
- Helps to establish the practice's mission and values
- Approves long-range plans and the annual budget
- Ensures quality of medical care
- Monitors performance against plans and budgets
- Reviews resource distribution

Other responsibilities of the board may include:

- Providing and monitoring institutional goals
- Interacting with other leaders in the community

In medical groups, most members of the board are physicians. Because their duty is to the group as a whole, they must put their own interests or the interests of their specialty aside and make the needs of the entire group their priority.

In most cases, board membership occurs via an election, with rules that are specified in the bylaws of the organization. It is imperative that the group's bylaws be properly adopted and that the procedures outlined in the bylaws are followed carefully. Failure to correctly follow the process could result in a challenge to the legitimacy of the process and invalidate actions under state law.

The board's prospective members need to be evaluated based on their ability to meet predetermined criteria that have been communicated clearly. At least annually, the board should conduct a self-review of performance and provide feedback to each of the board members. This should include a checklist of board responsibilities. Evaluation of present board members could include the following:

- Board members must meet the attendance requirement. This is usually a high percentage of all meetings (e.g., 75%).
- Board members must come prepared to meet and discuss the agenda items.
- Board members should be evaluated on their expertise. What skill is each specific member asked to contribute? Is the member an expert in business operations, finance, marketing, or law? It is not uncommon for the group's legal counsel to attend board meetings. At least in theory, board meetings can be protected by attorney-client privilege when legal counsel is present.
- Board members must respect the confidentiality of the board's activities. They must also support the decisions of the board outside the boardroom.
- Board members must disclose conflicts of interest.
- Board members must show respect to management and its role to implement board policy.
- Board members must act in a prudent manner, provide fiduciary responsibility, and understand their behavior is representative of the group at all times.

Medical groups are beginning to behave more like traditional business corporations. As part of this change, groups are adding outside persons to the board to improve the governance process and to bring in new ideas and perspectives. These individuals must be chosen carefully with consideration of a number of important criteria, including:

- A general understanding of the region, its business climate, political environment, and some of the key community drivers, as well as some perspective on healthcare and what is happening in the broad view
- Strategic thinking
- Willingness and ability to attend meetings
- Ability to treat information discreetly
- Previous experience as a member of a board
- No conflicts of interest or the appearance of such conflicts (e.g., not someone seeking to do business with the clinic)
- General business acumen
- Ability to contribute without dominating the board
- A history of working well in a group setting (i.e., a "good fit")
- Willingness to sign a confidentiality or nondisclosure agreement
- Willingness to accept fair compensation if applicable

Although many not-for-profit healthcare organizations do not pay their board members, the trend in the healthcare industry is to offer compensation, which can vary according to the size of the organization. Some large hospitals might pay board members as much as $20,000 annually for attending monthly meetings, while others offer much smaller amounts. In general, though, healthcare organizations are recognizing that it is acceptable and fair to offer some compensation in order to attract highly qualified and motivated board members.

The medical group's board must deal with a number of stakeholders in the quest to provide effective governance of the group. Some of these stakeholders are:

- Physicians in the medical group practice
- Other physicians in the community
- Employees
- Patients, their families, and caregivers
- Payers
- Government agencies at the federal, state, and local levels
- Hospitals and other healthcare entities
- Community members

An essential element of governance is the delegation of tasks and duties for the group. The principal governing body may decide, as allowed or even required by the group's bylaws, to develop a committee structure that addresses operational concerns and processes within the practice in conjunction with the administration. This is a great way to provide physician input in a structured manner instead of on an ad hoc basis. It also provides a great opportunity to develop future leaders by educating them in the committee process. Some of the more common committees within the governance structure are:

- Executive
- Finance
- Personnel
- Technology
- Quality review
- Management (usually in smaller groups)
- Research
- Recruiting
- Continuing education
- Managed care
- Strategic planning
- Medical practice development (i.e., growth)
- Operational performance
- Ad hoc committees for many purposes, such as new construction, service-line development, patient satisfaction, and contract review

Going through the process of creating the executive committee must include approval from a majority of stakeholders. It is doubtful that this type of change will be unanimous, although that is certainly preferred. Even though the concept is formally approved, board members will look for ways to revert back to the old form of governance. The executive committee should be consistent and firm and remind the board that this change was approved by the shareholders and there is an expectation of support.

Executive committee responsibilities include operational, financial, and board-assigned tasks, as well as preparing the agenda for and running board meetings.

Daily operational issues can be dealt with in the following ways:

- The healthcare executive will keep the executive committee informed about personnel, financial, or operational issues. Decisions regarding these issues shall be made by the executive committee, healthcare executive, or brought to the board, as appropriate.
- The healthcare executive or the executive committee may establish ad hoc committees for special projects, such as recruiting.

The executive committee oversees the financial health of the medical group practice by:

- Focusing on financial opportunities for the medical practice (both revenue enhancement and cost reduction)
- Approving annual operating and capital budgets
- Overseeing compensation plans and benefits
- Assessing and recommending investments in new programs and services
- Developing and managing debt strategy

- Recommending the timing and amount of quarterly shareholder bonuses to the board of directors

Governing needs to be concerned with the focus of group activities. Activities need to be grouped with consideration for function and customer interaction. In addition, leadership must be empowered to implement and act upon the governing board's policies and decisions. Typically, this would mean the group should focus on three areas of oversight:

1. Internal functions
2. External functions
3. Operations

Regular reports to the board, as well as benchmarking these activities, can be very useful for the effective governance of the organization. It is also important to understand how these activities interact. This interaction has to be governed carefully to prevent a silo mindset, or group think, from emerging.

Outside of the governing board, the top leader of any medical practice or healthcare organization is the executive officer. The purpose of the executive officer is to ensure the practice or organization operates efficiently, employees have the resources they need, and to ensure quality of care to patients. In short, the executive officer works to ensure the needs of the organization and its patients are met. Additionally, the executive officer provides:

- Leadership
- Support
- Representation
- Organization

Today, there is an increasing demand for healthcare executives and a decreasing pool of qualified candidates. This is primarily due to the number of healthcare networks and large corporate entities that require more leadership at higher levels. In order to compete with larger entities, smaller practices will need to make sure they are providing competitive career opportunities. In some cases, practices may need to hire a professional and provide them with education and additional experiences needed to become the executive the practice needs. The practice may wish to hire a professional recruiting firm for the top executive positions. Recruiting firms often have a wider range of candidates to choose from, can advertise more effectively, and have the experience to vet applicants.

Whether using a recruiting firm or not, the practice should consider the following when searching for an executive:

- The candidate's education
- The candidate's career experience
- The candidate's professional skills

Executive officers should have a thorough knowledge of and experience in the healthcare environment. Although unique in many ways, healthcare is still a business, and executives must be familiar with finance, marketing, and public relations. It is important that healthcare executives understand office politics among providers, staff, health plans, hospitals, and the community. Communication skills can make or break a healthcare executive. It takes talent and skill to be the liaison between the governing board, employees, and community.

It is every employee's responsibility to ensure clinic compliance with federal, state, and local regulations. It is the executive who will be held responsible by the governing board, and also the name on record for the regulating agencies. Executives must be skilled at determining the strategy of the organization and ensuring that the mission acts as the beacon for decision-making and business processes and outcomes. It is the combination of these skills that will determine the financial stability of the organization.[9]

It is the board's responsibility to provide such refinement through regular feedback sessions. Each year, the Harvard Business Review releases a list of the top 100 CEOs. Over the years, performance measures have evolved to include metrics beyond just finances, and also include relationships with employees, customers, suppliers and their communities. Graham Kenny says, "measuring performance is measuring relationships."[10]

The executive should work with the board of directors to define operating metrics to be used to evaluate the business health of the practice. Basic metrics would include practice growth, profits, productivity, staff retention rate, and patient satisfaction. The strategy should be defined and then reviewed to determine the effectiveness of the implementation. These key performance measurements should be written in objective terms and be specific, measurable, achievable, relevant, and time bound (SMART). These performance measures will be evident by the data and outcomes. The expectations should be clearly identified and defined prior to the review.

More subjective measurements will include evidence of relationships with people, both internally and externally. It is important for board members to speak with staff, patients, suppliers and community members to get a sense of the relationship skills that the executive demonstrates.

Many practices have failed not because the finances were at risk, but because staff, patients, and community members did not have a good experience with the practice. The problems could be anything from lack of leadership to systems that prevent patients from being seen in a timely manner to the clinic furniture looking dated or worn. All of these issues fall under the scope of executive leadership. Therefore, the board of directors should hold the executive accountable for such relationships and perspectives.

Just as employees should have regular feedback sessions with leadership, so should the board provide feedback to the executive. Although executive leadership should provide frequent feedback sessions, it is reasonable for the board to only provide feedback sessions twice per year, with one of those being the formal annual performance review. The review should be provided in a planned and private discussion. In most cases, a board subcommittee is responsible for conducting the review, with the chair providing the formal feedback. Reviews should include both the strengths and weaknesses, with a plan of expectations set forth for personal development for the next review period. Some organizations want a self-evaluation completed as well, and then a plan would be developed to bridge the gap. It should be an expectation that a healthcare executive will provide a professional development goal every year. The stronger the leader, the stronger the organization will be as a whole.

Corporate records are legal documents that must be maintained in accordance with pertinent state and federal laws and regulations, which may vary by state and jurisdiction. Accordingly, it is essential that the governance plan address retention, storage, and retrieval policies for business documents.

The primary responsibility for ensuring proper storage and retention should include a designated backup custodian if the process owner (e.g., the healthcare executive or physician owner or partner) is unavailable. The plan should also include a loss control process for electronic backup of important documents, such as partnership and shareholder agreements, employment contracts, equipment leases, and real estate records. Under most circumstances, it is prudent to retain a copy of important documents at a location physically distant from the primary storage location. This should prevent any type of disaster from destroying executed copies of significant information.

Many organizations keep original documents for the length of the statute of limitations pertinent to the most likely allegations related to the document. Some records are evergreen, whereas others may be replaced by newer versions. Examples of records include articles of incorporation, bylaws, employment agreements, medical records, and physician credentials.

Organizational culture is an extremely important aspect of medical practice governance. Of course, positive cultures need to be maintained, and any negative culture needs to be converted to a more positive one. Culture can be maintained by a focus on those aspects that are desirable. Recording the history of the group can enhance positive culture maintenance and make its accomplishments known.

Publishing the history of the group in newsletters and websites can help instill pride throughout the organization and maintain a positive culture.

Like policies and procedures, bylaws are dynamic documents that require regular maintenance. Changes in corporate law may require amendments to the bylaws, so a general review of corporate documents should be completed at least annually, with special attention being paid to those areas that may have been the subject of changes during the year. The following questions should be considered as the bylaws and policies of the group are reviewed:

- Has the group changed any committee structures this year?
- Has the group changed any of its procedures on elections?
- Has the group added any new shareholders or have any departed? If so, was their stock exchanged according to the bylaws?
- Are the duties outlined for officers and directors still current?
- Are minutes of meetings recorded, and was a quorum present when decisions were made?

- Were the key decisions made according to the bylaws and governance documents?
- Does the group do things differently today than it did in the past?
- Has the makeup of the governance changed enough to warrant reviewing a change to the bylaws?
- Has state corporate law changed since the group's bylaws were last reviewed by legal counsel?

Executives must protect the integrity of the bylaws, because failure to act within the scope of the bylaws may cause legal action by aggrieved shareholders and unnecessary intergroup relationship concerns. It is wise to periodically review the requirements of the bylaws with the board, so the board members fully understand them. It is essential that new board members be oriented to understand this material, and all applicable stakeholders must have access to the governance documents for reference.

SAMPLE QUESTIONS

1. **Establishing mission and vision, and setting strategic goals, fiscal management, and operational oversight is the responsibility of the:**

   A. Practice owner

   B. Administrative team

   C. Board of directors

   D. Physicians

2. **What is one advantage of being a nonprofit organization?**

   A. Income taxes are lower

   B. Property taxes are lower

   C. Payroll taxes are lower

   D. State taxes may be lower or exempt

Answers: 1-C, 2-D

TASK 3: ORGANIZATIONAL POLICY AND PROCEDURES

Organizational policies and procedures standardize practice operations. They are essential in providing clarity when dealing with issues that are critical to practice operations (e.g., human resources, operations, health and safety protocols, legal liabilities, and regulatory compliance).

Policies and procedures often are discussed together; however, they are not the same or equal. Policies are thought of as an overview, the information that helps staff make decisions. Policies provide guidance. Procedures are the various processes and steps that explain how to execute the policy. Put another way, policies are the overarching viewpoint of the organization and procedures set the policy in motion.

Policies and procedures should be written specifically enough to provide guidance and set organizational expectations, but broadly enough to provide managerial flexibility. A well-written and documented policy or procedure assists in compliance from a regulatory and legal perspective. Policies, since they are broader, will change infrequently, while procedures could change within months of finalizing or after staff members receive training.

KEY TERMS

Policy: The overarching viewpoint of the organization.

Procedure: Sets the policy in motion.

Written policies and procedures establish a standardized practice to reduce variation. If a policy and the procedure for executing it are accurate, helpful, and truly provide clear instructions, this naturally creates a more efficient and evolved workplace. Due to its very nature of explanation and information, it will set staff expectations. These documents serve as a resource for staff, particularly new staff, and create accountability for all. Well-written policies and procedures that are easily accessible also level the playing field for all staff members by reducing the necessity to remember all of the details of each policy and procedure.

Moreover, policy and procedure manuals serve as communication tools with your employees and leadership team. When a particular policy or procedure is not documented well, it will be realized quickly and can be adjusted. These overviews and directives are the unified place your employees can go to gain knowledge, information, and direction.

These policies and procedures, in whatever format they are shared, help to create compliance in a variety of ways. The explanation of how the practice sees the policy and clarifies its execution through the procedure provides an interpretation of the rules and requirements. This helps the employee understand both the policy and the importance of following the procedure. Multiple policies or procedures may intersect and work together as a unit to meet the requirements of different regulatory and accreditation bodies. This is a double-edged sword, though; if the policies and procedures are not well-written or defined, or if the information is incorrect or inaccurate, this can lead to problems with regulatory and accreditation agencies. It is important to regularly review all policy and procedure manuals, and keep them updated as necessary or appropriate.

Before any part of these documents is drafted, appropriate and relevant research must be conducted. If a committee or small group is drafting the policy, that group should be prepared to defend their viewpoint and research. Those who will utilize the policy or procedure should be consulted with and take part on the committee to ensure accuracy and efficacy. The committee should confirm that all regulatory information is up to date and applicable.

The writing of policies may prove difficult and challenging for some, while others may have very clear viewpoints and communication styles. The key to writing a strong policy and procedure is to be clear and direct. There is no need for flowery language or an overabundance of descriptive words or prose. Policies should be clear-cut written documents that relay the necessary information to all staff members who need it.

Once the documents are drafted, have the appropriate user groups vet the information for suitability and relevance. The healthcare executive should invite other leaders in the practice, as well as in some cases an outside consultant or legal representative, to review them. At the very least, the practice compliance officer should always review and approve policies and procedures to make sure they comply.

The elements of a well-written policy and procedure include but are not limited to the items below:

- Effective date, version, revision dates
- Title
- Purpose and scope
- Applicability
- Organizational goal(s)
- Definitions or glossary
- Duties of providers and staff — who is involved
- Operational procedures and detailed process
- Related policies or resources
- Policy review period
- Approvals
- Disclaimer that the policy and procedure may be revised without notice

The medical practice should have policies and procedures that accurately reflect the work completed in the practice. Depending on size, coordinate the policies and procedures based on work product, department or overarching goals. The departments most likely to have their own policy manuals are:

1. Billing and receivables
    - Contracted services

- In-house services
- Time frames
- Training

2. Human resources
    - Background checks
    - Conflict resolution
    - Drug screening
    - Education
    - Grievance procedure
    - Harassment prevention
    - Health examinations
    - Hiring
    - Immigration policy and I-9s
    - Legal compliance
    - Licensure
    - Onboarding and orientation
    - Performance evaluations
    - Skills assessment
    - Training

3. Patient care
    - Complaint procedure
    - Legal compliance
    - Patient dumping
    - Philosophy
    - Standard of care
    - Surveys

4. Inventory management
    - Assessment
    - Bids
    - Logistics
    - Procurement
    - Review periods
    - Stock levels and fulfillment
    - Types

5. Maintenance
    - Contracted services

- Equipment maintenance
- Preventive maintenance
- Repair schedules

6. Operations, including front and back office
   - Customer service
   - Scheduling
   - Training
7. Physician practice
   - Auxiliary staff
   - Bonus programs
   - Credentialing
   - Hospital programs
   - Peer review
   - Recruitment
   - Travel programs
8. Safety
   - Drills
   - Injury and illness prevention plans
   - Licensure required for staff
   - Safety protocols

The goal of clear-cut policies and procedures is to communicate how the practice operates and to ensure compliance with all federal, state, and local regulations. The responsibilities and expectations of employees should be given clearly so each staff member understands them. This allows employees to grasp how policies and procedures relate to their jobs, healthcare outcomes, and how to approach their individual tasks as well as a team's tasks. The policies and procedures are the only way for governing agencies to view the practice objectively. Well-documented, well-written, and up-to-date policies and procedures that are accessible to all employees is fundamental to the success of a medical practice.

SAMPLE QUESTIONS

1. The primary goal of establishing policies and procedures is to:

A. Gain executive buy-in

B. Create compliance

C. Hold employees accountable

D. Establish the organization's culture

2. It is important to regularly review all policy and procedure manuals and to keep them:

A. Filed

B. Secure

C. Updated

D. Private

Answers: 1-B, 2-C

ORGANIZATIONAL GOVERNANCE QUIZ

1. A sole proprietorship is defined as a business with a:

A. Single owner that is not established as a separate entity

B. Group of providers who share a space

C. Group of primary care providers

D. Single physician who has filed as a professional corporation

2. The board of directors of a medical practice is responsible for:

A. Engaging key stakeholders in the community and local government

B. Hiring and firing employees

C. Signing paychecks

D. Managing the day-to-day operations of the practice

3. When developing the practice's mission statement, it is important to include input from stakeholders:

A. Inside and outside the practice

B. At all organizational levels

C. Including patients and their families

D. Within the government

4. ________ cultures are hard-driving and focused on delivering high shareholder value, competing for capital and market share, fast decision-making, and the consistent delivery of on-time results.

A. Adhocracy

B. Clan

C. Hierarchy

D. Market

ANSWERS

1-A. A sole proprietorship is a business owned by a single individual, not a corporation. B and C are not business types. D would not qualify as a sole proprietor if the person has filed as a corporation.

2-A. Among its other responsibilities, the board of directors is responsible for engaging key stakeholders in the community and local government.

3-B. It is important to include input from stakeholders at all organizational levels when developing the practice's mission statement.

4-D. A market culture is hard-driving and focuses on competing for market share and results. Adhocracies are externally focused and adept at adapting to change. Clan cultures rely on personal relationships and collaborations. Hierarchies emphasize efficiency and standardized processes.

Notes

1. Kennedy, Allan and Terrence Deal. *Corporate Cultures: The Rites and Rituals of Corporate Life*, Cambridge: Perseus Books Group, 2000.
2. Drucker, Peter, The Leader to Leader Institute. *The Five Most Important Questions You Will Ever Ask About Your Organization*, San Francisco: Jossey-Bass.
3. Schein, Edward. *Organizational Culture and Leadership, Hoboken*: John Wiley & Sons, Inc., 2017.
4. Dewar, Carolyn and Doucette, Reed. "Culture: 4 keys to why it matters," http://mckinsey.com/business-functions/organization/our-insights/the-organizationblog/culture-4-keys-to-why-it-matters, March 27, 2018.
5. Craig, William, "The Importance of Having a Mission-Driven Company," *Forbes*, May 15, 2018.
6. Kolomiyets, Tetyana, "Organizational culture and its mission, vision and values," *UNECE Statistics Wikis*, last modified April 23, 2020, https://statswiki.unece.org/display/SCFP/Organizational+culture+and+its+mission%2C+vision+and+values; Jaruzelski, Barry, John Lehr, and Richard Holman, "The Global Innovation 1000: Why Culture is Key," strategy+business, Winter 2011, https://strategy-business.com/article/11404?gko=62080.
7. Chassin, Mark R. and Jerod M. Loeb, "High-Reliability Health Care: Getting There from Here," *The Milbank Quarterly*, September 13, 2013.
8. Quinn, Robert and Kim Cameron, *Diagnosing and Changing Organizational Culture: Based on the Competing Values Framework*, San Francisco: Jossey-Bass Publishing, 2011.
9. "Executive Job Descriptions." MGMA, http://mgma.com.carrer-pathways/foremployers/job-descriptions/executive-job-descriptions, 2020.
10. Kenny, G., "Create KPIs that reflect your strategic priorities." *Harvard Business Review*, Feb. 2020.

Printed in the USA
CPSIA information can be obtained
at www.ICGtesting.com
CBHW080207221124
17684CB00004B/17

9 781568 290607